Nursing and Mental Health Care

An introduction for all fields of practice

Transforming Nursing Practice series

Transforming Nursing Practice is the first series of books designed to help students meet the requirements of the NMC Standards and Essential Skills Clusters for degree programmes. Each book addresses a core topic, and together they cover the generic knowledge required for all fields of practice. Accessible and challenging, *Transforming Nursing Practice* helps nursing students prepare for the demands of future health care delivery.

Core knowledge titles:

Series editor: Dr Shirley Bach, Head of the School of Nursing and Midwifery at the University of Brighton

Communication and Interpersonal Skills in Nursing (2nd edn)	ISBN 978 0 85725 449 8
Contexts of Contemporary Nursing (2nd edn)	ISBN 978 1 84445 374 0
Health Promotion and Public Health for Nursing Students	ISBN 978 0 85725 437 5
Introduction to Medicines Management in Nursing	ISBN 978 1 84445 845 5
Law and Professional Issues in Nursing (2nd edn)	ISBN 978 1 84445 372 6
Leadership, Management and Team Working in Nursing	ISBN 978 0 85725 453 5
Learning Skills for Nursing Students	ISBN 978 1 84445 376 4
Medicines Management in Adult Nursing	ISBN 978 1 84445 842 4
Medicines Management in Children's Nursing	ISBN 978 1 84445 470 9
Medicines Management in Mental Health Nursing	ISBN 978 0 85725 049 0
Nursing Adults with Long Term Conditions	ISBN 978 0 85725 441 2
Nursing and Collaborative Practice (2nd edn)	ISBN 978 1 84445 373 3
Nursing and Mental Health Care	ISBN 978 1 84445 467 9
Passing Calculations Tests for Nursing Students	ISBN 978 1 84445 471 6
Patient and Carer Participation in Nursing	ISBN 978 0 85725 307 1
Successful Practice Learning for Nursing Students (2nd edn)	ISBN 978 0 85725 315 6
What is Nursing? Exploring Theory and Practice (2nd edn)	ISBN 978 0 85725 445 0

Personal and professional learning skills titles:

Series editors: Dr Mooi Standing, Principal Lecturer/Enterprise Quality Manager in the Department of Nursing and Applied Clinical Studies, Canterbury Christ Church University and Dr Shirley Bach, Head of the School of Nursing and Midwifery at the University of Brighton

Clinical Judgement and Decision Making in Nursing	ISBN 978 1 84445 468 6
Critical Thinking and Writing for Nursing Students	ISBN 978 1 84445 366 5
Evidence-based Practice in Nursing	ISBN 978 1 84445 369 6
Information Skills for Nursing Students	ISBN 978 1 84445 381 8
Reflective Practice in Nursing	ISBN 978 1 84445 371 9
Succeeding in Research Project Plans and Literature Reviews for Nursing Students	ISBN 978 85725 457 3
Reviews for Nursing Students	ISBN 978 0 85725 264 7
Successful Professional Portfolios for Nursing Students	ISBN 978 0 85725 457 3
Understanding Research for Nursing Students	ISBN 978 1 84445 368 9

BEBC Distribution, Albion Close, Parkstone, Poole, BH12 3LL. Telephone: 0845 230 9000. Email: learningmatters@bebc.co.uk. You can find more information on each of these titles and our other learning resources at **www.learningmatters.co.uk**. Many of these titles are also available in various e-book formats; please visit our website for more information.

Nursing and Mental Health Care

An introduction for all fields of practice

Steven Trenoweth, Terry Docherty, Joseph Franks and Reuben Pearce

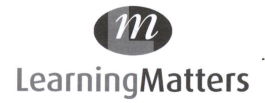

LearningMatters

First published in 2011 by Learning Matters Ltd

British Library Cataloguing in Publication Data

A CIP record for this book is available from the British Library

ISBN 978 1 84445 467 9

This book is also available in the following ebook formats:

Adobe ebook ISBN: 978 1 84445 785 4
ePub ebook ISBN: 978 1 84445 784 7
Kindle ISBN: 978 0 85725 033 9

Cover and text design by Toucan Design
Project management by Diana Chambers
Typeset by Kelly Winter
Printed and bound in Great Britain by Short Run Press, Exeter, Devon

Learning Matters Ltd
20 Cathedral Yard
Exeter EX1 1HB
Tel: 01392 215560
E-mail: info@learningmatters.co.uk
www.learningmatters.co.uk

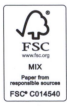

FSC
www.fsc.org
MIX
Paper from
responsible sources
FSC® C014540

Contents

Acknowledgements

The authors and publisher would like to thank the following for permission to reproduce copyright material:

Rethink Mental Illness (www.rethink.org) for profile on pages 45–6.

Every effort has been made to trace all copyright holders within the book, but if any have been inadvertently overlooked the publisher will be pleased to make the necessary arrangements at the first opportunity.

The publishers and authors would also like to thank Dr Steven Pryjmachuk, Senior Lecturer, University of Manchester and Thomas Beary, Senior Lecturer – Mental Health, University of Hertfordshire, for their very helpful feedback on early drafts of this book.

About the authors

Dr Steven Trenoweth is a mental health nurse and principal lecturer at the University of West London. He is responsible for teaching a range of health related topics at both undergraduate and post graduate levels specifically within the field of mental health and psychology. His interests include positive health and psychosocial interventions.

Terry Docherty has been a senior lecturer in mental health for nearly twenty years, and is currently working at the University of West London with a clinical link with the Central North West London Trust. His main areas of work include the delivery of the pre-registration programmes leading to the Advanced Diploma or BSc in Higher Education in Mental Health Nursing. His interests are in teaching in the areas of personality disorder, psychosis and legal and ethical issues in mental health nursing.

Joseph Franks is a mental health nurse and a lecturer of mental health at the University of West London. He is responsible for teaching a range of mental health topics and delivering this to students of mental health nursing, including the delivery of post registration qualifications in Psycho-Social Interventions for Psychosis. His interests include Family Interventions for Psychosis, Relapse Prevention Work and Early Interventions for Psychosis. He has a background of working within the clinical area of Intensive Rehabilitation often with service users who have serious mental illnesses; this provided him with the opportunity to develop his skills when working with this client group delivering Psycho-Social Interventions for Psychosis.

Reuben Pearce is an experienced mental health nurse and independent prescriber who has worked for Berkshire Healthcare Trust NHS Foundation Trust for the past fifteen years. Since qualifying as an RMN in 2002 he has experienced working in Assertive Outreach, inpatient services, A&E Liaison, Dual Diagnosis and Crisis/Home Treatment. Reuben has recently taken up a full time post as lecturer at at the University of West London, specialising in the pre registration mental health nursing programme and other post registration courses such as Non-Medical Prescribing and Psychosocial Interventions for Psychosis. Reuben is also a member of the Oxford Psych Course Team who provide training across the UK and in Hong Kong for psychiatrists in preparation for the Clinical Assessment of Skills and Competencies (CASC) Exam – part of the MRCPsych examination for the Royal College of Psychiatrists.

Wasiim Allymamod is currently working as a qualified nurse in a Forensic Service of a London mental health Trust. He qualified from the University of West London with a first class honours degree in Mental Health Nursing in 2008. He has recently been seconded to work with the psychology team and specialist work here includes working with treatment of people with a history of sex offending and fire setting. His interests are cognitive behaviour therapy and psychosocial interventions.

Introduction

This book examines the nursing care of people who are experiencing mental ill health regardless of field or clinical context. This is in keeping with future nursing care, which will require a more holistic approach (NMC, 2010a). The book explores the nature and meaning of mental health and ill health and how we can understand and respond to the needs of people experiencing mental distress. In so doing, we will explore the policy context for mental health care while helping you to clarify your own views about mental health and ill health, and how you may, in turn, improve your own mental health.

Book structure

Chapter 1: Understanding mental health and ill health

In this chapter we explore the various ideologies and paradigms that seek to explain the aetiology of mental ill health and how these in turn affect care processes and treatment interventions. In addition to the medical model, social and recovery models of care will be discussed along with various psychological approaches (such as behaviourism, psychoanalysis and so forth). This chapter will help you to understand and consider the nature of mental distress and help you to apply this knowledge to your own field and with different client groups.

Chapter 2: Clarifying your own personal values and beliefs

This chapter highlights the importance of clarifying one's own personal values and beliefs as a precursor to caring for the person in mental distress. A full discussion will be offered relating to interpersonal dynamics and belief systems that can hinder the development of therapeutic nursing relationships. The chapter will include a number of values clarification exercises and will explore the nature of values-based practice and the requirements for the delivery of compassionate care that seeks to respond meaningfully to the needs of patients.

Chapter 3: The policy context for mental health care

The provision of mental health care in primary care and community services has continued to develop and grow alongside more specialist inpatient, child and adolescent, substance misuse and forensic services. In this chapter we give you an overview of the most important policy frameworks to have emerged in recent years and their impact on modern mental health care delivery and nursing practice. Particular attention will be paid to the *National Service Framework for Mental Health*. This chapter also seeks to explore ways in which people with mental health problems may be socially excluded by communities and society, and the policy response to reducing stigma and disability.

Chapter 4: Mental and physical care needs

There is currently a much greater awareness of the poor physical health care that people in mental distress experience. This applies to both those with psychiatric diagnoses and also those with physical health problems whose related psychiatric difficulties may have an important bearing on ultimate treatment outcomes and the trajectory of their illness. This chapter seeks to explore the importance of being able to adequately meet both the physical and mental health needs of people in mental distress.

Changes to the role of the nurse in recent years will be discussed as well as how the nursing profession can provide holistic care in diverse settings. An overview of essential nursing skills will also be highlighted in providing holistic care for the client in mental distress.

Chapter 5: Legal and ethical issues in mental health nursing

This chapter offers an overview of the Mental Health Act 2007 and mental capacity. Importantly, it challenges the reader to consider the nature of morality and how differences in lifestyle choices may be misconstrued as psychiatric pathology. It also gives an overview of ethical principles and dilemmas in mental health care and encourages the reader to use best available evidence, ethical principles, and NMC standards and guidance to offer possible resolutions to complex cases such as consent.

Chapter 6: Communicating and relating

This chapter explores the importance of engaging with the person who experiences mental distress and how effective communication, active listening and strategies for relating can support the development of therapeutic alliances. Essential skills of communication and fundamental counselling strategies will be explored.

Chapter 7: Assessing mental health needs

Here, the various means of assessment of will be explored – from the use of structured frameworks (such as the ICD-10 medical taxonomy), through the semi-structured and unstructured interviews and screening for common mental health problems. The importance of attempting to understand the person's internal frame of reference and capturing personal narratives will be discussed, along with the need for comprehensive, holistic assessments of health and social care needs.

Chapter 8: Helping the person with mental health needs

In this chapter various strategies that could be employed by the nurse to help and support the person in mental distress will be discussed. This ranges from general supportive care through to more structured 'psychosocial interventions'. Experiential activities will be provided throughout and the particular emphasis on this chapter will be developing skills of helping.

Chapter 9: Improving your own mental health

In this chapter, the reader is invited to consider their own mental health and how this may be developed and enhanced. A discussion of stress vulnerability will be made and also the notion of life events and ambient stress. The notion of adaptive and maladaptive coping will be explored along with Copeland's 'Wellness Recovery Action Planning'.

Requirements for the *NMC Standards* and the Essential Skills Clusters

The Nursing and Midwifery Council (NMC) has established standards of competence to be met by applicants to different parts of the register, and these are the standards it considers necessary for safe and effective practice. In addition to the competencies, the NMC has set out specific skills that nursing students must be able to perform at various points of an education programme. These are known as Essential Skills Clusters (ESCs). This book is structured so that it will help you to understand and meet the competencies and ESCs required for entry to the NMC register. The relevant competencies and ESCs are presented at the start of each chapter so that you can clearly see which ones the chapter addresses. There are *generic standards* that all nursing students, irrespective of their field, must achieve, and *field-specific standards* relating to each field of nursing; i.e. mental health, children's, learning disability and adult nursing. Most chapters have generic standards, and occasionally field-specific standards are listed. This book includes the latest standards for 2010 onwards, taken from *Standards for pre-registration nursing education* (NMC, 2010a). Please visit the website for the book at **www.learningmatters.co.uk/nursing**.

Learning features

Activities

Throughout the book you will find activities in the text that will help you to make sense of, and learn about, the material being presented by the authors.

Some activities ask you to reflect on aspects of practice, or your experience of it, or the people or situations you encounter. *Reflection* is an essential skill in nursing, and it helps you to understand the world around you and often to identify how things might be improved. Other activities will help you develop key skills such as your ability to *think critically* about a topic in order to challenge received wisdom, or your ability to *research a topic and find appropriate information and evidence*, and be able to make decisions using that evidence in situations that are often difficult and time-pressured. Finally, communication and working as part of a team are core to all nursing practice, and some activities will ask you to carry out *group activities* or think about your *communication skills* to help develop these.

All the activities require you to take a break from reading the text, think through the issues presented and carry out some independent study, possibly using the internet. Where appropriate, there are sample answers presented at the end of each chapter, and these will help you to understand more fully your own reflections and independent study. Remember: academic study will always require independent work; attending lectures will never be enough to be successful on your programme, and these activities will help to deepen your knowledge and understanding of the issues under scrutiny and give you practice at working on your own.

You might want to think about completing these activities as part of your personal development plan (PDP) or portfolio. After completing the activity write it up in your PDP or portfolio in a section devoted to that particular skill, then look back over time to see how far you are developing. You can also do more of the activities for a key skill that you have identified a weakness in, which will help build your skill and confidence in this area.

Chapter 1
Understanding mental health and ill health

Steven Trenoweth

NMC Standards for Pre-registration Nursing Education

This chapter will address the following competencies:

Domain 1: Professional values

2. All nurses must practise in a holistic, non-judgmental, caring and sensitive manner that avoids assumptions, supports social inclusion; recognises and respects individual choice; and acknowledges diversity. Where necessary, they must challenge inequality, discrimination and exclusion from access to care.

5. All nurses must fully understand the nurse's various roles, responsibilities and functions, and adapt their practice to meet the changing needs of people, groups, communities and populations.

Domain 2: Communication and interpersonal skills

4. All nurses must recognise when people are anxious or in distress and respond effectively, using therapeutic principles, to promote their well-being, manage personal safety and resolve conflict. They must use effective communication strategies and negotiation techniques to achieve best outcomes, respecting the dignity and human rights of all concerned. They must know when to consult a third party and how to make referrals for advocacy, mediation or arbitration.

5. All nurses must use therapeutic principles to engage, maintain and, where appropriate, disengage from professional caring relationships, and must always respect professional boundaries.

6. All nurses must take every opportunity to encourage health-promoting behaviour through education, role modelling and effective communication.

Domain 3: Nursing practice and decision-making

2. All nurses must possess a broad knowledge of the structure and functions of the human body, and other relevant knowledge from the life, behavioural and social sciences as applied to health, ill health, disability, ageing and death. They must have an in-depth knowledge of common physical and mental health problems and treatments in their own field of practice, including co-morbidity and physiological and psychological vulnerability.

continued overleaf . . .

continued . . . . •••

3. All nurses must carry out comprehensive, systematic nursing assessments that take account of relevant physical, social, cultural, psychological, spiritual, genetic and environmental factors, in partnership with service users and others through interaction, observation and measurement.

4. All nurses must ascertain and respond to the physical, social and psychological needs of people, groups and communities. They must then plan, deliver and evaluate safe, competent, person-centred care in partnership with them, paying special attention to changing health needs during different life stages, including progressive illness and death, loss and bereavement.

7. All nurses must be able to recognise and interpret signs of normal and deteriorating mental and physical health and respond promptly to maintain or improve the health and comfort of the service user, acting to keep them and others safe.

Domain 4: Leadership, management and team working

4. All nurses must be self-aware and recognise how their own values, principles and assumptions may affect their practice. They must maintain their own personal and professional development, learning from experience, through supervision, feedback, reflection and evaluation.

NMC Essential Skills Clusters

This chapter will address the following ESCs:

Cluster: Organisational aspects of care

9. People can trust the newly registered graduate nurse to treat them as partners and work with them to make a holistic and systematic assessment of their needs; to develop a personalised plan that is based on mutual understanding and respect for their individual situation promoting health and wellbeing, minimising risk of harm and promoting their safety at all times.

By the second progression point:

ix. Undertakes the assessment of physical, emotional, psychological, social, cultural and spiritual needs, including risk factors by working with the person and records, shares and responds to clear indicators and signs.

By entry to the register:

xii. In partnership with the person, their carers and their families, makes a holistic, person centred and systematic assessment of physical, emotional, psychological, social, cultural and spiritual needs, including risk, and together, develops a comprehensive personalised plan of nursing care.

> **Chapter aims**
>
> By the end of this chapter, you should be able to:
>
> * describe how nurses, regardless of their specialist fields, can understand the mental health of their patients;
> * understand the use of terminology in describing mental ill health;
> * highlight various models and theories of mental distress;
> * consider unifying framework(s) for understanding mental distress.

Introduction

In this book we consider the impact of mental ill health on the well-being of individuals. Assisting people to achieve a state of overall well-being is undoubtedly an important goal of nursing care. In our attempts to assist people to overcome adversity that might be affecting the mental health of people we care for, we must understand the nature of mental distress. This is the starting point of the nursing care process – we need to understand the patient's experience and needs before we can intervene and provide care. This is often very complex.

You might think that mental health issues are the responsibility of mental health nurses who specialise in the care and treatment of people who experience mental distress. However, as we shall see in this chapter, the nursing profession as a whole is moving towards delivering more **holistic** care, and there are expectations that all nurses, regardless of field, will be able to respond to the mental health needs of their patients. In the same way, mental health nurses must be able to respond to the health care needs of their service users, whether they are children, whether they have a co-morbid physical illness, or whether they have a mental health problem and a learning disability.

In this chapter we will first explore the different meanings that may be attributed to mental health and mental ill health. This is important as, regardless of the field of nursing you are studying, you will encounter many perceptions about mental health and mental ill health in your studies and in practice, and you will come to realise that how one perceives a phenomenon is often related to how one responds to it. We will explore what using terminology means, before looking broadly at what mental health and what mental ill health is. We will then explore the various theories and models of mental health and ill health, and look at the complex relationship between them, and how a holistic viewpoint can help all nurses, regardless of their field, to help patients to improve their mental health.

Clarifying terminology

As we have already touched on in the introduction, the words that we use in our lives can be a subtle way of communicating perceptions and biases. Words can act as symbols for a larger set of often otherwise unstated assumptions and ideologies. Look at the example given in the case study.

Case study

Sandra is a service user with a long history of schizophrenia, which has had a devastating effect on her life. She is often very angry with mental health services, which she feels do not always meet her needs. She has complained that she feels she is not involved in her care. Sometimes she breaks off all contact. Unfortunately this has meant that she has been hospitalised six times in the last four years. Sandra manages to do some voluntary work in a local Age Concern charity shop when she feels able. She would like to find more permanent work but says she has been unlucky in finding a position. She is a qualified primary school teacher but would be willing to undertake any work. At present she is receiving state benefits. Recently, things have been difficult for her as she is struggling with the break-up of a long-term relationship.

Sandra has been diagnosed with diabetes and is being seen by a diabetic nurse specialist with whom she recently had an argument. She felt that the nurse specialist 'kept going on' about her diagnosis of schizophrenia, which Sandra feels has nothing to do with her diabetes.

Sandra is also under the care of a community psychiatric nurse (CPN) with whom she has a good relationship. Sandra relates the argument she has had with the nurse specialist:

'She kept telling me I am mentally ill. She said "Because you are schizophrenic you need to remember to take your diabetes medication." I asked her what she meant and she got defensive. She thought I was stupid. I asked if she was mentally healthy. I don't know what good mental health is and she didn't seem to know either.'

In this case study, Sandra asked what seem to be straightforward questions: What do you mean by mental illness? What is mental health? The concepts of *mental health* and *mental illness* are terms that are value laden – that is, they are imbued with more meaning than can be found by a dictionary definition. Such terms carry with them a set of personal, social and cultural assumptions. Sandra, for example, felt that the nurse specialist saw her as 'stupid' because of her mental health issue.

Activity 1.1 — *Reflection*

Think for a moment and jot down any words you associate with the term *schizophrenia*.

- What does the term imply to you?
- How did you develop your ideas about the term? That is, where do you get your ideas from?
- What other terminology do people sometimes use to describe people who experience mental ill health? What effects might this have on individuals?

An outline answer is given at the end of this chapter.

You might have thought that the term **schizophrenia** was a *mental illness* or a *diagnosis*. You might have even jotted down the term *madness*. You might have assumed that people with this diagnosis are dangerous or violent, or that they need long-term institutional care. It can be quite difficult to reflect on where our assumptions come from. Often they are transmitted by our parents, friends and siblings. Sometimes the media (books, magazines, newspapers as well as film and television) represents and reinforces a particular view about groups of people.

Symbolic interactionism is a sociological theory that seeks to account for such socially constructed ideas (Haralambos and Holborn, 2008). Put simply, the theory suggests that people construct their own social reality through culturally meaningful symbols such as words, uniforms, flags, social interactions and gestures. While such symbols can give people a sense of common identity, they can also lead to stigmas and stereotyping that can often go unchallenged. In nursing care it is vital that we are aware of such symbols and that our culturally imbued and socially constructed knowledge does not affect the quality of care that we provide.

In this book we use the broader terms *mental health problems, mental ill health* or *mental distress* as symbols that encompass the experience of all people with psychological difficulties rather than words that are medically bound, such as *mental illness* or *mental disorder*, which may convey or reinforce the view that mental health problems have a biological or psychiatric origin – as we shall see later, there are indeed many different interpretations of mental health and mental distress.

For this reason, the *Working in partnership* review (DH, 1994) suggested that the nurses who care for people with mental health problems should not be called *psychiatric nurses* but *mental health nurses*, to reflect the diverse nature of their work and to ensure they are not tied exclusively to a medical framework for their practice.

Furthermore, we must be careful to avoid the trap that may be laid by our culturally imbued ideas (see Chapter 3). For example, we must not assume that an individual's problems centre solely on a medical diagnosis. This is called 'diagnostic overshadowing' where one diagnosis or condition is given pre-eminence over other health issues (Jones et al., 2008). Take, for example, a child who has been diagnosed with, and is receiving treatment for, cancer. This is very likely to be a time of considerable stress and distress for the child and their friends, siblings and parents. However, the nursing and other health care staff may be focused on treating the cancer and may not recognise or respond to the potentially long-lasting psychological distress experienced by the child and their friends and family. As such, nurses of all fields must recognise that anyone can experience mental distress, regardless of whether or not they have a diagnosed mental illness, and it is the duty of the nurse to provide holistic support to the person in need.

What is mental health?

Before continuing our journey exploring mental distress it is useful to pause to consider what is meant by *mental health*.

Activity 1.2	*Reflection*

What do you believe to be the essential features of mental health? Do you consider yourself to be mentally healthy?

An outline answer is given at the end of the chapter.

The World Health Organization (WHO, 2010) defines mental health as:

> *a state of well-being in which the individual realises his or her own abilities, can cope with the normal stresses of life, can work productively and fruitfully, and is able to make a contribution to his or her community.*

Health is, also, the WHO argued in 1946, *not merely the absence of disease or infirmity* (WHO, 1946). The WHO's definition of health and mental health takes a broad view, seeing it as a reflection of our ability to function, cope within and make a contribution to society. This reflects the social nature of our functioning as human beings.

It is important to realise that one does not *have* mental health – one has a *personal sense* of one's own mental health. The WHO's definition recognises this when it states that mental health is the *realisation* of one's abilities and so forth. It is not, therefore, something that can be assigned by others but a personal and 'subjective' experience. We are mentally healthy when we believe it, when we sense it, when we see ourselves behaving in mentally healthy ways. However, we must understand, of course, that there are times when a person may feel mentally well and may not be aware of problems that may be evident to others. For example, a person who experiences an unusually elated mood with high energy levels and who may become irritable and angry may be seen by others as having a mental health problem, such as mania.

What is mental illness?

Activity 1.3   *Critical thinking*

The use of the term 'illness' when describing mental health problems carries with it many implications. Take a few moments to think about and note down what is generally implied by the term 'illness'.

An outline answer is given at the end of the chapter.

Did you note down that an 'illness' is a disease arising from a germ or infection, or some physiological problem within the body? If so, you might argue that an illness implies a medical or biological problem associated with some form of bodily dysfunction. Now if we were to apply this to the concept of mental ill health, we might assume that mental health problems have a biological basis arising from some form of anatomical defect or physiological dysfunction within the brain.

When we talk of a mental 'illness' we are, technically, talking of a mental health problem that has been assigned a psychiatric diagnosis (psychiatry is the branch of medicine that diagnoses and treats mental disorders). There are two main medical diagnosis systems (or taxonomies) that are currently in use: the WHO's *International classification of diseases and related health problems* (*ICD-10*), (WHO, 2004); and the American Psychiatric Association's *Diagnostic and statistical manual of mental disorders* (*DSM-IV*, APA, 2000). Both these systems attempt to catalogue mental disorders by assigning a diagnosis based on an assessment of symptom clusters. For example, if one is experiencing unpredictable attacks of severe anxiety with sudden onset of palpitations, chest pain, choking sensations, dizziness, and feelings of unreality, with fear of dying, losing control, or going mad, then a diagnosis of *panic disorder*, using the *ICD-10* classification system, may be warranted.

Case study

Brenda is a 28-year-old housewife and formerly a registered child nurse. She spent many years working with sick children and specialised in intensive care. She is very proud of her nursing career and feels that she made an important contribution to people's lives.

Brenda is an articulate, intelligent woman who feels ashamed of her inability to cope. She has a child aged five and says that her panic attacks started soon after he was born. She is constantly worried, very anxious and unable to cope with looking after her child. When she has a panic attack she starts to tremble, her pulse races, she has chest pain and she feels dizzy and sick. The frequency and intensity of her panic attacks have been increasing recently to the point where they have become severe and disabling, leading to a functional impairment in her everyday life.

She says that things are out of control for her and she is at the mercy of her panic attacks. She feels she is a hopeless mother and that nothing she ever does is right. Her husband wants another child but she doesn't know how she is going to cope. She doesn't know what to do when she is in this state. She tries to keep it hidden from her husband who says she is just being 'silly'.

In this case study, we can see that Brenda is experiencing many of the key features of a *panic disorder* as defined by the *ICD-10,* namely anxiety, worry, feelings of being unable to cope and that things are out of control, experience of chest pain and dizziness.

There is evidence that seemingly links underlying biological dysfunction of the central nervous system with mental health problems. For example, chronic and enduring depression and stress, and post-traumatic stress disorder can lead to damage of the brain, particularly the hippocampus, amygdala and frontal cortex (Perna et al., 2003). Depression may result from physical trauma to the brain where the ability of the brain to transmit information is disrupted (Brown, 2004). Some degenerative brain diseases such as Alzheimer's have clear organic aetiologies; for example, neuroimaging seems to indicate that people with Alzheimer's have neural tangles in their brains that appear to kill brain cells. Poor nutrition and diet have also been linked to mental health problems (Mental Health Foundation, 2006). For example, some nutrients such as folic acid, omega-3 fatty acids, selenium and tryptophan appear to reduce the symptoms of depression. Some infections that can affect the development of the foetus, such as prenatal influenza, can increase the risk of a diagnosis of schizophrenia in adulthood (Brown, 2006). There also appear to be heritability factors associated with many mental illnesses (Kring et al., 2010). Studies that attempt to capture the role of heredity typically explore the incidence of illnesses in families and among twins, assuming that if identical twins raised apart have similar rates, then this would suggest a genetic predisposition or vulnerability towards a particular disorder. For example, some twin studies suggest that identical twins are three times more likely than non-identical twins to develop schizophrenia if their twin also has this diagnosis (Kring et al., 2010).

Activity 1.4	*Evidence-based practice and research*

If you believe that mental distress has a biological origin and is thus symptomatic of psychiatric dysfunction and disorder, what sorts of treatments do you think might be offered?

An outline answer is given at the end of the chapter.

Look back at your notes from Activities 1.3 and 1.4. If you feel that mental ill health has a biological origin, you are likely to suggest a biological response, such as the prescription of psychiatric medication. The medical model claims that biological factors (such as the anatomy and physiology of an individual's nervous system and their genetic make-up) are crucial risk factors in the development of a mental illness (Engel, 1977). For example, an excess of the neurotransmitter *dopamine* has been linked to schizophrenia. Indeed, if one perceives that the root cause of a mental health problem is physical, then the treatment that is prescribed is likely to be targeted at a biological level, and as such the management of symptoms is likely to involve medical interventions, such as the prescription of medication, electro-convulsive therapy (ECT) or, in extreme cases, neurosurgery.

There are, however, some people who dispute that mental distress is an 'illness' or who suggest that the role of biological predeterminants of mental distress have been overemphasised. Assuming for a moment that there is clear agreement between people in terms of the diagnosis of a person's mental illness (Bentall, 2003 suggests that there is not), there is as yet no clear evidence to prove the connection between biological dysfunction and mental health problems. The interpretation of twin studies, for example, is not always clear, with some suggestions that findings of studies are based on a poor statistical analysis of results (Bentall, 2003), and there are few studies of twins being raised fully apart to provide conclusive evidence (Kring et al., 2010).

Engel (1977) argued that the biomedical model may restrict our understanding of health and illness in that it does not help us to understand how beliefs, expectations and hopes impact on the trajectory of health and illness. For example, when arriving at a psychiatric diagnosis the psychiatrist seeks to make 'objective' judgements about a person's mental state and mental capacity. There is, of course, a danger that a person will be seen solely in terms of their diagnosis – this is known as **labelling**. As we saw with Sandra, once such a label has been applied it can difficult to remove.

In fairness, however, people who subscribe to the biomedical model do not inevitably rule out the interaction of biological factors with, for example, the environmental experiences of an individual. Geneticists, for example, might argue that an individual has a *predisposition* to a particular illness but that environmental factors play an important role in whether this gene finds expression. Unquestionably, the medical model has offered much to people who experience mental distress and has helped many on their road to recovery, and we would be wise not to dismiss this approach. However, we must also remember that the medical model is one approach and that people experiencing mental distress should have available to them a range of options they can choose from to help them to meet their particular needs and wishes.

Other models and theories of mental ill health

There are many interpretations of mental ill health in terms of its origins (**aetiology**) and many forms of possible treatment. Perceptions of mental distress have changed over time, not only in terms of its aetiology but also in terms of how it is thought best to help subsequently.

In Activities 1.3 and 1.4, you explored the concept of illness and how biological understandings of illness might lead to medical treatment. In the next activity, you are asked to consider alternative views of mental ill health:

Activity 1.5   *Decision making*

1. How might different peoples or cultures see mental ill health differently?
2. How might societies' views of mental health and illness lead to the development of services?
3. What alternative explanations are there to account for mental ill health?

For each alternative explanation you can think of, try to think about how it might lead to alternative treatments for mental health issues.

An outline answer is given at the end of the chapter.

In answering the first question of Activity 1.5 you might have said, thinking back to the idea of symbolic interactionism, that people and cultures 'construct' meanings surrounding health and illness, and that some cultures have a scientific interpretation of health and illness while others rely on spiritual or lay beliefs regarding aetiology and treatment of ailments. For example, one culture may interpret a vision of Christ as a miracle; another may see this as a visual hallucination and a symptom of psychosis.

Individual clients therefore may have different interpretations of their own health and illness, and it is important to clarify this as it may be a barrier to progress. For example, lay theories of mental health may be at odds with views held by health professionals and with known scientific 'best available evidence'. Individuals may also hold unrealistic expectations with regard to achieving maximal physical or mental health. It is fair to say that, currently, mental health services in the UK are predominately medical and scientific in their outlook and that the medical approach is seemingly the predominant paradigm, but this belies the fact that there are many different interpretations, models and theories of mental distress. In answering the first question, you might have, quite correctly, thought that there are psychological and social factors that underpin mental health issues. It is to these alternative models of mental ill health that we now turn.

Psychological models

Broadly, the various psychological models and theories suggest that mental distress is underpinned by how one thinks and feels about oneself and the world and/or how one behaves. This in turn has an impact on how we feel about ourselves (such as our self-esteem, self-confidence and so on) and our confidence and our place in the world.

Behavioural models argue that we learn (or are 'conditioned') by our environment. **Behaviourism** is a branch of psychology that assumes that the behaviour of an organism may be changed (or 'conditioned') by environmental events (or 'stimuli'). There are two main theories: **classical conditioning** and **operant conditioning**. We acquire much of our learning through classical conditioning. For example, if you are hungry and smell your favourite food, you are likely to salivate. This was the basis of a study by Ivan Pavlov in the early twentieth century. Every time food was presented to a dog, a bell was struck. Over time, the dog would salivate when the bell was struck *before* the presentation of the food. The dog had learned to *associate* the sound of the bell with the presentation of the food. Classical conditioning is thought to be a mechanism by which people acquire phobias; this is based on work initially undertaken by Watson and Rayner in 1920 (Gross, 2010). Here is how it is thought to work: a person is exposed to a frightening situation (such as a loud noise or a disturbing event) that leads to a fear response, at the same time experiencing a neutral stimulus (that is, an object or event that would otherwise be non-threatening – a spider, for example). This neutral stimulus may then become associated with the fearful situation. Over time fear is experienced on the presentation of the neutral stimulus – the person has been conditioned to respond fearfully to the neutral stimulus.

Operant conditioning sees an important relationship between an action and its consequences – called the Law of Effect. This law suggests that an action that has good consequences will tend to be repeated, whereas an action that has bad consequences will tend not to be repeated. The stronger the association between a stimulus and a positive effect (that is, the strength of **positive reinforcement**) the more likely it is that the stimulus will condition one's behaviour.

BF Skinner (1965) suggested that our response to a stimulus tends to persist, and our response to the stimulus will survive even if, occasionally, it produces an unfavourable response. In addition to positive reinforcement (where favourable consequences are likely to strengthen an association between a stimulus and a response), Skinner also suggested that **negative reinforcement** (where a favourable response is associated with the termination of an unpleasant stimulus) is also likely to increase the frequency of a response. For example, one may learn to associate not opening a utility bill – which requires us to part with money we do not have – with temporary peace of mind. One may think: 'I don't have to worry about something I don't know about.' Similarly, not studying for an exam helps us to deal with exam anxiety – we ignore and avoid the reality of the exam. Both of these events help us to cope, but only in a short-term way. They are ultimately **maladaptive** and do not help us to cope in a positive way. The short-term relief of an unpleasant stimulus can lead to long-term consequences. Not studying for an exam may be tension relieving, but it will not help you to pass it. How might you condition yourself to develop more **adaptive** responses to exam anxiety? That is, how can you learn to associate exam revision with positive consequences?

Cognitive behaviour therapy (CBT) is another psychological approach that seeks to account for how our behaviours, thoughts and feelings underpin mental health problems. CBT is a structured approach used to treat a variety of mental health issues (such as depression, anxiety, phobias and pain problems). CBT assumes that what we think affects our emotions and behaviour. The approach is problem-oriented and is focused on resolving the factors that maintain difficulties rather than on the difficulties' own origins. It focuses on altering unhelpful thoughts or behaviours that may be contributing to the mental health problem. The patient learns to view their thoughts and beliefs about themselves and the world as hypotheses whose validity is open to testing.

Beck's (1976) *Cognitive therapy and the emotional disorders* provides the framework for contemporary CBT. Beck argues that our experience of the world led us to form assumptions or *schemata* about ourselves and the world, which are subsequently used to organise perception and to govern and evaluate behaviour. Sometimes these schemata may be untrue or unhelpful; they may be rigid, extreme and resistant to change, and are often sweeping generalisations about ourselves (e.g. 'I am bad') and the world ('I am worthless'). This, Beck argued, leads to depression and **negative automatic thoughts** that become more and more frequent and intense, and a vicious circle is formed.

Another historically very important psychological theory which seeks to account for mental distress is that of **psychodynamic** theory, stemming from the work of Sigmund Freud (see, for example, Freud, 2006). It is not possible for us to give a comprehensive overview of his complex theory (of which there have been many subsequent modifications made by later psychoanalysts). However, the essence of the theory states that mental distress is grounded in our early development. Problems that have not been satisfactorily resolved during our development may find expression in later life.

Social models

Social, sociocultural and interpersonal models argue that the basis of mental distress is grounded in the social world. This approach assumes that the way people feel and think is affected by the circumstances in which they live and work, which are in turn the product of economic and political conditions in society (Scottish Executive, 2005). For example, social stressors arising from job loss and unemployment, loss of a close friend, relative or spouse, stress from within the family, chronic social adversity (such as poverty), stigma, social exclusion and a lack of community acceptance and tolerance, lack of social support and isolation and a lack of a sense of belonging with a community can have a profound influence on our mental health (Holmes and Rahe, 1967; Bentall, 2003). The 2002 Office for National Statistics (ONS) survey of people with neurotic and psychotic disorders, alcohol use and dependence and drug dependence found that 33 per cent of people in this group were unemployed or economically inactive (ONS, 2002). The report also found that people with mental health problems often experienced a severe perceived lack of social support, were more likely to be single, divorced or separated, and were far more likely to be living in rented accommodation with a perceived lack of space (ONS, 2002).

Indeed, there is much evidence that social inequalities and social disadvantage are disabling and are risk factors that are likely to increase mental distress and/or contribute to relapse among those who already experience mental distress. For example, people who have been abused or the victims of domestic violence have higher rates of mental health problems. Prisoners in overcrowded environments have a high rate of mental health problems, such as suicide and self-harm (Howard League for Penal Reform, 2005). People with an identified mental health problem are more likely to be excluded from work; those with a common mental disorder are four to five times more likely to be unemployed, twice as likely to be on income support and four to five times more likely to be getting invalidity benefits, compared to the general population. Financial pressures are the most frequently cited causes of depression; people with mental health problems are more likely to be in debt, to be trapped in poverty and to have difficulties managing money than other members of the general population.

For Harry Stack Sullivan, mental health problems were reflective of social 'problems of living' (Sullivan 1968). Durkheim's *Suicide: a study in sociology*, first published in 1897, argued that suicide was a reflection of the degree of social integration that an individual experienced (Durkheim, 1997). Higher rates, he suggested, occurred when people were insufficiently integrated into social groups. Brown and Harris's seminal work *The social origins of depression* (Brown and Harris, 1978) argued that loss and the stresses and strains in women's daily experiences are implicated in depression. For example, ongoing, stressful social and interpersonal circumstances, such as longstanding difficulty in relationships, can lead to an increased likelihood of developing depression. Such vulnerability in women, Brown and Harris found, may be enhanced by having three children under the age of 14 years, by not working outside the home, by having no one to confide in and by the loss of one's mother by death or separation before the age of 11 years. For people with a mental health problem, their psychiatric diagnoses may be more than a way of classifying mental disorder. Some would argue that they add to the 'problems of living' of this group by acting as a label by which they are stigmatised, thereby reinforcing, perpetuating and even possibly justifying social disadvantage.

There are also wide cultural variations in the interpretation and perceptions of health and illness. In mental health, we can see this in cross-cultural research into depression and anxiety. For example, when presenting initially with depression Latin American people tend to report more bodily symptoms, whereas people in the USA and Western Europe have higher rates of reported headaches (Morrison and Bennett, 2006). There are also gender differences in the presentation of mental and physical health and illness. For example, men have a shorter life span and higher rates of physical health problems; they engage in more risk-taking behaviours that have a health impact (such as smoking, unprotected sex, unprotected exposure to the sun and so on) and have higher incidences of drug/alcohol use and suicide. Such health issues, it has been argued, are influenced by, and often seem to reflect, socialisation into particular gender roles where the male role may be culturally imbued with assumptions of social obligations and the apparent need to be strong, achievement oriented and competitive. Goldberg (1977) called this the 'bind' of masculinity; being a man may seriously damage your physical health and mental well-being – statistically at least (Trenoweth and Lynch, 2008).

What are considered to be 'good' mental health, mental ill health and the cultural presentation of symptoms of mental ill health are therefore relative judgements, and definitions of what is mentally healthy can change across time, across cultures and between individuals, based on socialisation and one's own personal experience. Sometimes, of course, the opinions of others about our mental health may differ from our own personal judgements.

Recovery and positive health models

Recovery and positive health models have been gaining much ground recently. They take a different stance to the medical, psychological and social models in that their starting point is how the individual may be assisted to achieve a life that is personally fulfilling to them, recognising strengths, assets and abilities, rather than focusing on disabilities, deficits and symptoms.

Recovery approaches draw a line between **complete recovery** – in which an individual returns to their level of functioning before they experienced mental ill health – and **social recovery** – which focuses on helping the person *towards* recovery, and involves an emphasis on social support, realistic planning, significant working relationships, encouragement, appropriate treatment, choice and self-management (Warner, 1985; Matthews 2008). In the later case, much emphasis is placed on the ongoing process of *recovering* from mental health problems. Here, an emphasis is placed on supporting the person with an aim to improving their overall quality of life despite the presence of 'psychiatric symptoms'. Hence, recovery in this sense:

> *is not about regaining a problem-free life – whose life is? It is about living life more resourcefully, living a satisfying and contributing life, in spite of limitations caused by a continuing vulnerability to disabling distress.*
> (Watkins, 2001, p45)

The recovery approach has found expression in the *Guiding statement on recovery* (NIMHE, 2005b). The statement sets out the principles and values of recovery focused care, which involves changing the orientation and behaviour of nurses and mental health services from a negative focus on an 'illness', condition or circumstance to helping people to rebuild, reclaim and take control of their lives.

Guiding statement on recovery (NIMHE, 2005b)

Recovery-oriented systems of care will:

- focus on people rather than services;
- monitor outcomes rather than performance;
- emphasise strengths rather than deficits or dysfunction;
- educate people who provide services, schools, employers, the media and the public to combat stigma;
- foster collaboration between those who need support and those who support them as an alternative to coercion;
- through enabling and supporting self-management, promote autonomy and, as a result, decrease the need for people to rely on formal service and professional supports.

In July 2009, the Future Vision Coalition (a group of UK-based charities and mental health organisations) set out a new vision for mental health. It argues for a broader, public health approach and sees that good mental health is important for an overall good quality of life. In this sense, mental health is an issue for everyone in society. It argues for effective positive mental health promotion to be a policy priority for the UK government that includes building resilience and targeted prevention work with 'at risk' groups and individuals and in areas such as prisons, schools and workplaces.

Positive health approaches take this notion of recovery one step further. They assume, as Martin Seligman (2002, p xi) puts it, that people *want more than just to correct their weaknesses*; they want to live a life imbued with personal meaning and happiness. In this sense, Seligman (2002) argues that happiness is not the hedonism of momentary pleasures but *authentic* and enduring happiness where one recognises and plays to one's signature strengths. Typically, in helping people to find such happiness the starting point is not on deficits but on strengths, such as wisdom and knowledge; courage; humanity and love; positive relationships with communities; temperance; and transcendence (strengths that help to connect people to something larger than themselves, such as aesthetic appreciation, a sense of purpose and spirituality) (Seligman 2002). For Seligman (2008, p15), the focus on positive health *is not only desirable in its own right . . . it is likely to be a buffer against physical and mental illness.*

Mental ill health as a complex phenomenon

Mental ill health is a complex phenomenon and as such it is not likely that any one approach will account for the various dimensions of an individual's experience. As our knowledge and understanding of mental health and mental ill health increases, there will inevitably be a rethink about how the various parts of the jigsaw fit together. As such, there will continue to be a need for various diverse theories and models that seek to account for an individual's experience (and extensions or revisions to existing ones) and a variety of interventions that individuals may wish to draw upon to support their recovery.

In this sense, there is no correct model or one theory that can stand as 'truth' when we attempt to understand the totality of an individual's experience of mental distress (Engel, 1977; Trenoweth and Price 2008). In fact, each of the models we have explored focuses on different aspects of human functioning and helps us to understand different aspects of experience. Potentially, therefore, the models and theories are *complementary*, and taken together they can develop our understanding of an individual's distress and open up many different and varied avenues of care and treatment. This point was stressed by Engel in 1977 when he proposed a **biopsychosocial model** of disease. Here Engel argued that a purely biomedical approach to mental distress was limiting and that there is a need to explore how psychological and social factors combine with the biological to affect the trajectory of illnesses. Engel (1977) was arguing that there is a need to include the *person* as well as the illness in developing an understanding of their health problems. Likewise, also in 1977, Zubin and Spring were arguing for a *new view of schizophrenia* that sought to explore how stressors could lead to a breakdown of coping in people vulnerable to schizophrenia. They assumed that people have a degree of vulnerability to schizophrenia that is *inborn* (for example, genetic factors and the 'internal environment' of the individual) and *acquired* (for example, the influence of traumas, perinatal complications and life events) that, due to the interaction and presence of certain circumstances, will challenge and provoke a crisis for a person's mental health. Zubin and Spring (1977) argue that such challenging circumstances ('exogenous stressors') include life events stresses – such as bereavements, marriage and divorce – that require a degree of coping and readjustment in the person's life. In vulnerable people, there may be a failure to cope and adapt to such stresses that may place their mental health under strain and increase the likelihood of mental ill health or relapse.

It might be tempting to think of *mental ill health* or *mental illness* as the exact polar opposite of *mental health* – that is, that one either 'has' mental health or mental illness, as if they were discrete categories to which one is assigned. However, it is more fitting to see mental health and mental illness as existing on a continuum; as such one may experience *degrees* of mental health (and mental distress), and this varies and fluctuates at various times in our lives. One of the ways in which our mental health might fluctuate might be as a response to the amount of stress that we experience in our lives. Indeed, it seems that we as individuals can vary in response to exposure to stress as Zubin and Spring (1977) suggested above. In this sense there is no 'us' and 'them'. There are not 'mentally ill people' as a distinct or separate group but all of 'us' who can, and do, experience varying degrees of mental health and mental distress.

A more holistic view sees mental health as encompassing not only such social factors but also physical, psychological, emotional and spiritual dimensions of self. As such, the model is an attempt to *pool the wisdom from all of the models* (Zubin and Spring, 1977, p109). Swinton's holistic model has five inter-connected dimensions (Swinton, 2001).

- Physical (the biological aspect of our selves).
- Social (our relationships with others).
- Emotional (the way in which we feel about ourselves and our lives).
- Psychological (beliefs and perceptions that we hold about ourselves and others).
- Spiritual (the meaning that we attach to our lives).

Swinton's model suggests that our experience of health and ill health is likely to be multi-dimensional rather than one-dimensional. Importantly, as one dimension is affected this will impact on other dimensions of ourselves. This suggests that our physical well-being and our mental well-being are interrelated. For example, a problem with our physical health is likely to have implications for our social, emotional, psychological and spiritual well-being. Let us pause for a moment and consider this in more depth.

Activity 1.6   *Reflection*

Using the holistic framework above, spend a few moments reflecting on how cancer might affect our holistic well-being. That is, how might this disease affect our social, physical, psychological, emotional and spiritual dimensions of self?

An outline answer is given at the end of the chapter.

People with physical illnesses have comparatively high rates of mental health problems. In fact, there is considerable evidence that much psychological distress among people with various health conditions goes unacknowledged and is not recognised. Without such recognition the person in distress may not receive the help they need to support them at difficult times in their lives. As nurses we care for people in a variety of situations and contexts. People may experience co-morbid mental distress (that is, mental distress that exists concurrently with other health issues), and this may subsequently impact on the trajectory of both issues. For example, people who are depressed tend to experience pain more, which has an impact on both the trajectory and recovery from illness (Gureje, 2007). The key message here is that in order to understand the mental distress a person might be experiencing we must look at the whole person.

'Good' mental health, we may argue, can result only if each dimension is in harmony – that is, that we feel physically fit and able, that we make a valid and worthwhile contribution to the lives of others, that we feel positive about ourselves and our lives, that we hold ourselves in esteem and as a person of worth, and that we feel our lives have direction, purpose and meaning. However, this would seem to imply that people with chronic or long-term conditions cannot have good mental health. This is clearly not the case. But painful, debilitating and disabling health problems are more likely to undermine our subjective experiences of mental health and hence may lead to mental distress.

Look at the following case study.

Case study

John is 34 years of age, married with two young children. He experiences severe asthma attacks that have proved difficult to treat. This, and the fact he has no academic qualifications, has restricted his job opportunities.

John has recently been made redundant from his job as a forklift truck operator at a local timber merchant. His job was not very well paid, but it allowed him and his family to live a relatively comfortable life. Locally, there are no vacancies for people with his skills and as he has no other qualifications his job opportunities appear quite bleak. Before long the redundancy money was used up to meet bills. John has begun to wonder how he can provide for his family. He feels it's his job to be the breadwinner – just like his father – but he is worried that he will be unable to meet their financial needs. He has begun to feel an unworthy husband and father. Increasingly it is difficult for him to get motivated, and his appetite is poor and his sleeping pattern is erratic. He appears sad and sullen and does not look after his personal hygiene. He doesn't want to leave the house, he says, and he doesn't want to socialise or talk to his friends. John tells his wife that they are better off without him.

John was admitted to hospital via casualty last night after having a very severe asthma attack. He is quiet and uncommunicative with nursing staff.

A cursory glance at the case study might suggest that John has experienced a severe asthma attack and that his quietness and uncommunicativeness are related to his fears over his physical health. His lack of personal hygiene may be construed as stemming from problems with mobility due to possible breathing problems. There may be a suspicion of an underlying chest infection that has exacerbated his asthma. However, how does a holistic understanding of John's current situation and experiences help us in our delivery of nursing care? By looking more holistically we can determine that in addition to his physical health issues, John is also experiencing significant issues in his psychological, social, emotional and spiritual dimensions of self. The loss of his job has added significant stressors to his life – particularly financial. His job prospects seem to be poor and he feels unable to provide for his family. This may have implications for how John sees his role within the family and may have an impact on his masculine identity. It appears that John is experiencing some symptoms of depression. As such, our holistic understanding of John's mental and physical health issues, while adding a dimension of complexity, ultimately can reveal more useful insights and a targeted response in terms of our nursing care.

Chapter summary

In this chapter we have looked at how terminology can affect our perceptions – and in particular our understandings of mental health problems. We have discussed how mental health and mental ill health may exist on a continuum; as such one may have *degrees* of mental health (and mental distress), and this varies and fluctuates at various times in our lives. We have also explored the various models and theories that have sought to account for mental distress (including the medical, psychological, social and positive health/ recovery approach). We have also explored a unifying framework for understanding the person, that of holism, as a way of appreciating the totality of the person's experience, including their mental and physical dimension of self, which may be of assistance to all nurses in discharging their professional duty of providing holistic care.

Activities: brief outline answers

Activity 1.1: Reflection (page 8)

The term 'schizophrenia' is technically a medical diagnosis that refers to a set of experiences where a person may experience delusions or hallucinations. It is often used incorrectly to imply a split personality. You may have been exposed to media representations of people diagnosed with schizophrenia and sometimes to attention-grabbing headlines. Nurses must be able to challenge this 'received wisdom' as it might have significant implications for care.

There are other terms that have, unfortunately, been used to describe people who experience mental ill health. Terms such as 'schizo', 'loony' and 'nutter' are not uncommon and can even be found in the popular press from time to time. Such terms are derogatory and often have very negative effects on the person to whom such labels are applied. They serve only to stigmatise a person and potentially isolate them from communities, which can have a dramatic effect on the person's progress towards recovery.

Activity 1.2: Reflection (page 9)

The World Health Organization (WHO) defines mental health as:

a state of well-being in which an individual realizes his or her own abilities, can cope with the normal stresses of life, can work productively and is able to make a contribution to his or her community. In this positive sense, mental health is the foundation for individual well-being and the effective functioning of a community.
(WHO, 2010)

In this sense mental health represents our ability to function in and be a part of our communities. The concept of 'well-being', mentioned in the WHO definition above, is often used to imply the totality of a person's health experience. By this we mean that well-being is often a holistic experience where a person feels both physically and mentally well and that their life is satisfying and has purpose and meaning. Another important aspect of the WHO definition of mental health is the ability to cope with the usual stresses and strains of life. This means that being resilient to some degree and being able to resolve life's problems are also important features of mental health.

Activity 1.3: Critical thinking (page 10)

Illness is poor health resulting from physical disease – a state of being sick. It often implies a biological dysfunction within the person's body. Other words associated with the term can include sickness, impairment, disorder, ailment and affliction. When we talk of 'mental' illness there is a danger that we may interpret mental health problems as being a disease or affliction. This rather assumes that the origins of mental health problems lie in the person's biology – that is, their anatomy or physiology. If we assume this to be the case, then it is likely that we would suggest treatments, such as medication, that seek to alter or change a person's biology. However, as we have discussed in this chapter, there are in fact many different models that seek to account for mental health issues (the social and the psychological, and so forth). Therefore, we must not assume that a person's mental health issue has a biological origin. This is why in this book we often use the term 'mental health problem' (as opposed to mental illness) to describe people's experience.

Activity 1.4: Evidence-based practice and research (page 12)

People who see a biological basis for mental disorder would most commonly prescribe a medical treatment such as medication, electroconvulsive therapy or, in extreme cases, neurosurgery.

Activity 1.5: Decision making (page 13)

Constructions of mental health and mental ill health are often socially determined and this changes over time. In fact, whether or not something is even considered to be a mental health issue is subject to change. Sometimes, cultures have alternative ways of viewing what we might perceive to be mental ill health, and their understandings may have supernatural or religious bases. It is clear that if a society believes in the medical basis for mental ill health, then it will fund medical services as a response. If it sees mental ill health in supernatural terms, hospitals will be irrelevant and alternative help and advice may be sought. In addition to the medical approach, there are also psychological and social models that seek to explain mental ill health.

Activity 1.6: Reflection (page 19)

Of course, there are wide individual variations in the response to any health issue but here you may have felt that cancer affects us as follows.

- Physical – pain, lethargy.
- Social – withdrawal from friends and family, seeking reassurance from friends and family, joining support groups.
- Emotional – anxiety, worry, stress, sadness, grief, fear.
- Psychological – thoughts about self and ability to cope, loss of control, thoughts that one is a burden.
- Spiritual – reflections on the future, reflecting on the meaning of the disease.

Further reading

Bentall, R. (2004) *Madness explained: psychosis and human nature*. London, Penguin.

An important book, if rather complex at times, which argues against the medical understanding of mental ill health. Bentall argues that mental illness labels such as schizophrenia are meaningless and criticises the medical approach to mental health care.

Chapter 2
Clarifying your own personal values and beliefs

Reuben Pearce

NMC Standards for Pre-registration Nursing Education

This chapter will address the following competencies:

Domain 1: Professional values

2. All nurses must practise in a holistic, non-judgmental, caring and sensitive manner that avoids assumptions, supports social inclusion; recognises and respects individual choice; and acknowledges diversity. Where necessary, they must challenge inequality, discrimination and exclusion from access to care.

5. All nurses must fully understand the nurse's various roles, responsibilities and functions, and adapt their practice to meet the changing needs of people, groups, communities and populations.

8. All nurses must practise independently, recognising the limits of their competence and knowledge. They must reflect on these limits and seek advice from, or refer to, other professionals where necessary.

Domain 4: Leadership, management and team working

4. All nurses must be self-aware and recognise how their own values, principles and assumptions may affect their practice. They must maintain their own personal and professional development, learning from experience, through supervision, feedback, reflection and evaluation.

NMC Essential Skills Clusters

This chapter will address the following ESCs:

Cluster: Care, compassion and communication

3. People can trust the newly registered graduate nurse to respect them as individuals and strive to help them to preserve their dignity at all times.

Cluster: Organisational aspects of care

9. People can trust the newly registered graduate nurse to treat them as partners and work with them to make a holistic and systematic assessment of their needs; to develop a

continued overleaf . . .

continued . . .

personalised plan that is based on mutual understanding and respect for their individual situation promoting health and well-being, minimising risk of harm and promoting their safety at all times.

14. People can trust the newly registered graduate nurse to be an autonomous and confident member of the multi-disciplinary or multi-agency team and to inspire confidence in others.

Chapter aims

By the end of this chapter, you should be able to:

*   identify how self-awareness is central to your ability to provide sound nursing care;
*   develop enhanced ability to communicate in difficult situations;
*   develop effective relationships through reflective practice;
*   explore how powerful your own value systems are and how they may influence your relationships with others.

Introduction

When you begin to consider working with people who are mentally distressed you may start to think – or even worry – about how you are going to manage. You may well start thinking: 'What on earth am I going to do if somebody starts to cry in front of me or becomes angry?' Imagine a scenario relating to somebody who is mentally distressed that causes you most anxiety; this will probably not be hard to do as it is likely to be at the forefront of your mind. If you *are* beginning to think like this, be assured that it is perfectly normal and healthy. It can be seen as positive because you are beginning to consider how you might manage yourself in a difficult situation.

When working with the mentally distressed, self-awareness is absolutely integral to your role as a nurse. Put plain and simply, if you are not aware of your own feelings and the effect of your behaviour on others, then you cannot be aware of other people's thoughts, feelings and behaviours (McCabe and Timmins, 2006). These are the themes that you are going to explore in this chapter as a cornerstone for effective nursing practice. You may start to realise here that your development as a nurse may go beyond the realm of a professional role into that of self-development. You may find that the development of the knowledge, skills and real-life experience associated with self-awareness will also see you grow dramatically as an individual in the wider context of your life. Learning to be a nurse may enhance your ability to be a parent, for example, where you also have to adopt a role in order to benefit others, in this case, your child.

Most nurses enter nursing for a reason. It could be, in part, linked to the likelihood of job security, a pension or the flexibility of working hours that can be achievable through nursing (Stein-

Parbury, 2005). Putting all practical reasons aside, you may well have reflected on what you feel you enjoy and have come to the conclusion that you have an interest in working with people. It is very likely that your interest in people is directly related to a desire to be of help to them. Having discovered that you enjoy and are quite good at working with people, you apply and join the nursing programme where you begin to work with patients and other health care workers. Throughout your nursing career you will be developing the ability to use yourself to guide you in your interactions other people. You will continually ask yourself questions, such as 'How has my patient just reacted to the way I communicated that piece of information? How would I feel if I was in his position? How would I behave?' You can use yourself to help guide your choice of actions, words and behaviour towards other people. In this way you will find yourself able to adapt to many different situations and people who may be very different to you in terms of how they think, how they act and what they believe (Hargie, 2006).

Through self-awareness you recognise and draw from past life experiences, current circum-stances, future hopes and expectations. You start to realise how they contribute to your feelings, attitudes, values and beliefs. These in turn affect what you do and what you notice about how you interpret other people's behaviour; in other words, it is only through self-awareness that you are able to clearly recognise your own values and beliefs, and begin to separate or identify how these may influence how you interact with patients (Underman Boggs, 2007a). These skills of understanding our internal and external reactions to what other people say, or how they behave, and also what you yourself say and do, are crucial to the helping relationships you will aim to build with people who are mentally distressed.

Activity 2.1   *Critical thinking*

With a friend, colleague or relative, identify something each of you believes in and is passionate about: it might be your favourite band or musician – or any subject.

Now ask the other person to try and convince you that you are wrong about your chosen subject because they feel their own chosen passion is far better.

- How did the discussion go?
- How did you feel about the way in which the other person put their argument across?
- Are they able to change your belief in your chosen subject?
- Are you able to appreciate how their chosen subject might mean something to them?

There is no outline answer to this activity.

Bear in mind how difficult it can be to try to impose your own thoughts about what you are passionate about on to somebody else, and keep that in the back of your mind throughout this chapter.

Becoming self-aware

Chapter 6 explores self-development in light of how you communicate and relate to others. It is, however, worth touching upon developing self-awareness here. The ability to become aware of your own behaviour and separate your own ideas, values and beliefs from those of your patient is something that will develop over a period of time (Howard, 2010). You will also find that even when you think that you have become skilled at the process you will still require some level of support developing it further. Nursing is a very rewarding and enjoyable career, but it can be very emotionally draining, as you will often find yourself face to face with the task of managing powerful raw emotions. Throughout both your student days and your career you should have plenty of opportunities to develop your self-awareness skills further through being encouraged to reflect on your practice with a view to building on your reflection/self-awareness for better interpersonal skills. You might describe this development as that of becoming a more insightful, wiser person.

If we break this concept of the 'self' down a bit further, we can consider the identity of the self, i.e. personal identity. Having a sense of self might be described as fundamental for being an adult person in that it is a major component in what shapes our personality (Sanders, 2003). The identity or self that we form as we become adults results from experiences that have occurred during childhood and through adolescence (McLeod, 2007). This is not the only theoretical perspective on the formation of the self, but it is a fairly good theory for understanding the concepts as applied to working with other people. Through this psychodynamic perspective, a person's identity is developed through interaction with others. For example, the ways other people act towards you can provide valuable information about the kind of person that you are. Your sense of identity – or at least parts of it – is always evolving in relation to what is happening in your life (Rungapadiachy, 2008).

Activity 2.2   *Reflection*

You might now think for a moment about how your identity has changed since commencing your nursing programme.

- Have you changed?
- Have your core values changed?
- What is it that guides you in what you do?

Some outline ideas on this activity are given at the end of the chapter.

The activity above may have led you to consider your belonging to the nursing profession as membership of a group. This sense of belonging to the nursing profession will have an influence over your sense of self, possibly as much as the role of nursing itself. Membership of different groups – for example the nursing profession, a karate club, a book club, following a particular fashion, being a festival-goer – will contribute to your sense of identity. As your group membership changes over the years, so will your identity. In part, you choose the groups you wish to belong to in order to determine your own identity. Consider teenagers, if you will, who start to rebel against the norms of their parents.

One way in which you might become immediately more aware of yourself is to give somebody feedback on how they have behaved.

Activity 2.3   *Communication*

Role-play with a trusted colleague a situation in which they play the role of a patient who has been very rude to you. You could start by playing out the scene where they are rude to you.

- Now try to feed back to your colleague how their behaviour has been, in a way that you consider respectful.
- Then ask for some feedback from the other person on what you have just said to them. How did it make them feel?

Sometimes it can be more powerful to record the role play so that you can watch yourself.

- Swap roles so you can be the patient too; this can be useful for better understanding a patient's perspective – in this case, why they have been rude.

There is no outline answer to this activity.

Now consider the sense of identity and individuality as it relates to the patient. Many factors will affect this: the nature of hospitals, the illness that the patient has, nursing procedures and other constructs that determine the way that nurses care for people who are unwell; all these things can play a part in removing a person's sense of identity and individuality (Underman Boggs, 2007a). This process of deindividualisation can lead to distorted behaviour. For example, a patient may act in a childlike manner, which can make you feel annoyed with the person and lead you to respond to them in a parental way. The parental response can reinforce the lack of individuality in the person (taken away by the hospital setting), thus further increasing the childlike behaviour (Diener, 1979). It is only through self-awareness that you might realise that you are potentially making a situation worse through your own annoyance with the childlike behaviour from the patient.

So we have seen that your sense of self has been developed and will continue to be shaped through your interaction with other people while at the same time directly affecting your interactions and their outcomes. This suggests that your social experience is fundamental to your sense of self, and vice versa (Kagan and Evans, 1995). It has been suggested that 'self' is both objective (the 'me' – derived from other people's attitudes and behaviour), and subjective (the 'I' – the individual's inner response to other people's attitudes). By taking on those attitudes of others towards yourself (the 'me'), the 'I' reacts (Mead, 1934). This capacity of people to be reflexive – that is, to be able to reflect upon aspects of themselves – is one of the things that makes people able to understand themselves and others (Cook, 1999).

Attitudes

We now move on to consider what attitudes mean to us. They might be seen as events or feelings that go on inside each and every person, including you, and these events might be difficult to identify without insight. These internal attitudes can be both positive and negative (Hargie, 2006). The feelings will most likely be directed towards an object, a person, a group or an issue – for example, 'I really like the lecturer who teaches us for Anatomy and Physiology', or 'I can't bear the way in which the ward sister arranges the off-duty', or 'I think that it is good to spend a minimum of ten minutes daily speaking to each patient on the ward'. These examples could all be seen as the voicing of attitudes by the person who is making the statements. It is true that people often have attitudes towards others but they also have attitudes towards themselves; and perhaps to make things more complex the attitudes they hold towards themselves will have a massive impact on their attitudes towards others. This may be what is happening in the following case study.

Case study

Jenny is a conscientious nurse working in the intensive care unit at the local hospital. One afternoon a patient she has spent a lot of time with, and whom she has been very kind and friendly to, is rather rude to her and says that she does not want to speak to Jenny any more. Jenny immediately feels very rejected and becomes quite frustrated by the attitude of this patient since she had spent a lot of time trying to engage her. Jenny decides that she is going to avoid speaking to that patient again for the rest of the shift.

Activity 2.4   *Critical thinking*

- What do you think is happening with Jenny in the case study?
- Whose needs are coming first?
- Do you think that Jenny is obstructing the interaction with the patient in any way through her own needs?
- How might you manage a patient who says they do not want to speak to you after you have invested a lot of time with them?

An outline answer to this activity is given at the end of the chapter.

Perhaps Jenny has a need to be liked by everybody and this was actually clouding her interaction with this patient. This is known as **perceptual filtering** (Stein and Parbury, 2005). Perceptual filtering is an unconscious process. It could be described as a lens that is placed on our mind that makes the world look a certain way. However, you might not be aware that it is just the filter causing the view. So long as the patient is being thankful in response to Jenny's kindness, Jenny accepts the patient. However, when the patient is no longer able to meet Jenny's needs by being kind in response, Jenny finds it painful and will no longer accept the patient.

It might be that beneath the friendly exterior Jenny presents to others as someone who has low self-esteem. She attempts to feel better by getting positive comments from patients.

If you have a strong positive attitude towards yourself, you will be seen as having a good sense of self-esteem, and perhaps you do generally feel pretty good about yourself. If you tend to think badly about yourself or even dislike yourself – that is, you have strong negative attitudes towards yourself – you might be described as somebody with low self-esteem. People who have high self-esteem will probably find that they are happier with their day-to-day lives and generally feel more confident most of the time (Stein-Parbury, 2005).

Do you often find yourself comparing how you feel and behave to how you see and believe others feel and behave? If you do, then this is perfectly normal and is one of the important ways through which people develop a view of their self. For example, think for a moment about somebody you really like or admire – do you wonder how you might be similar to that person or wish you were similar in more ways? Have you ever seen somebody behave badly and pondered to yourself 'Blimey, is that how I come across when I behave in that way?' You might then cringe at your own behaviour and feel embarrassed.

Consider a person or even a particular group of people whom you like or whom you aspire to be like. Both consciously and unconsciously you might find that you adopt some of the characteristics of that person or group. You may have noticed that people in a relationship, or people who are best friends, develop similar characteristics in their behaviour. Because of mutual respect and liking of each other's characteristics, people may adopt some of the attitudes displayed by that other person or group. This point demonstrates how attitudes that form part of the self are largely developed through comparison with others. The comparisons people make to other people are vital in shaping a person's sense of identity and self-esteem (Wosket, 2002).

Values and beliefs

Integral to the self are the values and beliefs that people hold. In order for a person to be their adult self they will have a set of values that they have formed through their experiences (McLeod, 2007).

Activity 2.5   *Reflection*

Make a note of how you might react to the following statements.

- I couldn't work with a paedophile; I would refuse to work with them out of principle. They should be executed, in my opinion.
- I will not put up with somebody using abusive and foul language in my presence – I would ask them to stop using such language because it is wrong.
- It is wrong that you attempted to kill yourself; life is too precious. God bless you, I will pray for you tonight and I will help you through this difficult time.
- I want to work with people as I like to make people feel better – I like to make people happier in their lives.

There is no outline answer to this activity.

It is difficult to say what is right or wrong about any of the statements in Activity 2.5. However, you might argue that each of these statements holds the values of the person making the statement. The values apparent in the statements may not reflect the values of the patient. The statements could then be viewed as demonstrating an attitude or belief and deemed judgmental by the patient. The statements could also be seen as imparting the values and beliefs of the nurse, thus overstepping professional boundaries. This might have a detrimental effect on rapport and thus a less than positive outcome for the patient.

When you are working with people who are mentally distressed, the values and beliefs you hold as a nurse can have a massive impact on how you react to any given situation, and this can have a direct impact on the experience and outcome for patients in many different ways (McCabe and Timmins, 2006). Your values and beliefs will guide your behaviour and can shape your attitudes (Bowers et al., 2009). Reflect back for a moment and think about what brought you into becoming a nurse in the very first place. If you think carefully, you may find that actually your reasons for embarking on a nursing career are rooted in your core personal values and beliefs.

Values may be described as *engrained views about what people consider to be ideal and the ways in which they go about achieving what they see as ideal* (Chambers and Ryder, 2009). A very obvious way of demonstrating this is through political parties; each political party holds a particular set of values at their core and strives to meet its objectives in a way that is in keeping with those values. Political groups may attract people with slightly differing personal values, but people pick a party that is closest to their own personal ideals. It is clear, therefore, why people may feel betrayed when political parties or individual politicians do not hold true to the core values they claim to support.

The core values that you hold may be few, but they make up a set of values that are central to your personal and moral sense of being. Core values help guide people through good and bad times during their lives (Maslow, 1999). Values will also play a part in a person's cultural and sub-cultural identities. For example, consider musical tastes; one person may listen to Dubstep and another to Emo rock. This choice may well be rooted to some degree in values that have been generated or linked to the individual self.

You could argue that sometimes we need to behave in a way that to some extent conflicts with our own personal values and beliefs because of the needs of somebody else (Rogers, 1980). This can create some internal conflict and you have to make a judgement call on yourself. An extreme example might be a survival situation whereby a vegetarian decides to eat some meat and also offer meat to their child in order to prevent them both dying from starvation. The bigger 'core value' to the parent is ensuring their child stays alive. Equally, some people may be willing to die in order to stay true to their values and beliefs, for example, through defending their people or country through war. This can go further still to killing other people to demonstrate their values and/or force them on to others. These examples highlight the sheer power of emotion that values generate in a person; they also demonstrate how important it is to be aware of the impact of your own values and beliefs and those of the people with whom you work. A nursing example is the situation where the mother of newly born twins refuses a blood transfusion because of her religion and she dies. What do think about this situation and how does this make you feel in relation to your own values?

Through developing an acute awareness of your values, you should find that you are better able to consider what is and what is not acceptable to you in terms of the situations you find yourself in as a nurse. Have you ever felt very strongly about a person's behaviour and felt the need to challenge that person? How might you manage a situation where you believe somebody is acting in an unpleasant manner towards a patient? Would you feel the need to confront and report that person? You might feel so strongly that you do not care whether challenging the behaviour has a detrimental effect on the relationship that you have with that person. When you feel that your values are being compromised, you may find that everything else is less important than standing by those values (Edwards, 2009).

Activity 2.6   *Critical thinking*

Be as honest as possible in how you answer these questions.

- What are your spiritual beliefs?
- What are your political beliefs?
- Where did these beliefs come from?
- What impact do you think these beliefs have on your views regarding your role in helping others?
- If you were to fully adopt your political and spiritual beliefs into your role in helping people, how might you behave? Would there be any difference?

If you feel comfortable discussing these ideas, make a note of your responses to the questions above and take them into a session with your colleagues for further exploration. It is likely that strong feelings will be evoked when you talk about your beliefs. What were the reactions from others when you shared your beliefs? Were there any strong negative or positive reactions? This is a good way of testing out some of the themes we are discussing in this chapter.

There is no outline answer to this activity.

It is important to remember and be aware that when values are challenged, people can become very defensive, aggressive or despondent because values are rooted in the core of people's personalities (Howard, 2010). You have to be very careful about how you approach challenging people; you can read more about challenging people in Chapter 6 on communicating and relating.

Values bring consistency to people's behaviour, and give them a sense of personal and cultural identity. Values can and will act as a guide on how people think, feel and behave. In the same way that you might follow guidelines or instructions to build a model, you might argue that values are your own personal guidelines on how to behave and thus provide consistency to your behaviour. A child who has not fully formed their personality and identity to their full will not know how to cope or behave in certain situations and will need parenting in order to be contained and not run riot. Values are highly resistant to change, but change in values is possible, and when a change does occur in a person, then it will have an impact on how they behave (McLeod, 2007).

At this stage it might be worth offering some clarification regarding beliefs, which are similar to values but not the same. You might want to consider beliefs as opinions or ideas that are linked to values, from which attitudes are developed.

Values → beliefs (opinions, ideas) → attitudes

Figure 2.1: How values can shape attitudes

As already discussed, values and beliefs are very resistant to change, so throughout history there have been wars all around the world in relation to religious, political and cultural beliefs (Egan, 2010). It will take a profound experience for a person to fundamentally change one of their beliefs. For example, you might have heard of a person who has had a near-death experience and has therefore decided to do something completely different with their life, or of somebody who has witnessed a terrible outcome of following one of their beliefs, which has led them to question that belief and see things differently.

Presenting yourself

Would you agree that you have a private self and a public self? It is highly likely that you present yourself in public differently from the way you might in private. Consider Facebook for a moment and how people present themselves using certain photos and language. Or consider how you might behave differently towards your grandparents than you would in front of your friends when down at the pub. If you think this is true, consider why this might be. Could it be that you want to project a certain image of yourself to people on Facebook? Could it be that you are respecting the values and beliefs held by your grandparents through your respect for them as individuals who care about you?

People present themselves in many different ways to different individuals and groups, often for good reason. Would it be appropriate for a police officer to reveal to a suspect he was about to arrest that he believes in ghosts and goes ghost hunting at the weekends? People take care to present their 'public' selves in ways that give different information to different groups of people (Goodman and Clemow, 2008).

Now think about this from the patient perspective. If the patient is feeling very sick, unwell and unhappy, then they are presenting you with that image of themselves. They might be trying to demonstrate their level of sickness or, quite the opposite, they may be trying to play down their level of sickness. It can therefore be difficult to find out what is really going on for a person while they are immersed in presenting themselves in a certain fashion (Moss, 2008). The way a person presents themselves is likely to be because of their situation, and their wish to have different characteristics or to be in a different situation. An example would be a man who is depressed but holds values and beliefs that it is 'not masculine' to talk about your worries.

This is where key communication and assessment skills are paramount in your role as a nurse. These skills are needed to break down such barriers for the patient in the safest possible way emotionally, in order to help them on their road to recovery.

Activity 2.7 — Communication

This is a role-play activity needing a minimum of three people.

- Person 1 will be trying to convince Person 2 to go out to a nightclub with them as they are in the mood for a party.
- Person 2 does not want to go because there will be people there they don't want to see and they have to work the next day.
- Person 3 is carefully observing the interaction between the other two.

You should try to get your own way for about five minutes before finishing the role play. Once you have finished, don't say anything to each other; just write a few thoughts in response to the following questions.

- How did you feel within yourself?
- What did you think of the other person in this interaction?
- How do you think the other person perceived you?
- What do you think influenced the feeling you had towards the other person?

The observer will also note down their thoughts about how the two people in conflict conducted themselves.

- Now compare notes – are the perceptions as you expected?

An outline answer to this activity is given at the end of the chapter.

Now think about these observations and the themes discussed within this chapter and observe how different people (including yourself) cope in conflictive situations in practice.

It is important to remember that being able to reflect and think about how you present yourself to others does not mean you have to be constantly objectively self-aware, for example when at home on your own. You will almost certainly be self-aware in the subjective sense most of the time, such as when considering what you want to eat or what you want to wear, or how you feel (Kagan and Evans, 1995). This is about being aware of your internal thoughts and feelings. However, it is unnecessary to spend the whole time being introspective – you would make yourself depressed. This is why it can feel so good to sometimes not have to think about anything, particularly when you are outside your working role – you need to find time to relax.

Objective awareness may come about through an event that makes you aware of how other people might see you (Kagan and Evans, 1995). Becoming too objectively aware in the extreme sense can lead to self-consciousness that can lead to anxiety and depression – as mentioned above. A healthy bit of objective self-awareness can help you to adapt the things that you say and do to improve how you do them. In your role as a nurse this is where you should aim to be.

You may now have established how you might present different facets of yourself depending on the situation you are in. You can consider this adaptation further in the next activity.

Activity 2.8   *Reflection*

Think about different ways through which you might be objectively aware while at work on a busy ward and make a note of them. Examples might be:

- catching a glimpse of yourself in the mirror when you are washing your hands;
- rereading a report that you have written that the ward sister will be reviewing later in the day.

In these examples and those that you have noted down for yourself, the underlying question that you may be raising is 'Is this how I am going to appear to other people?'

There is no outline answer to this activity.

You are likely to become objectively self-aware if you feel you are being watched or examined, such as when the ward sister reads your report or a patient's relative is watching you redress a wound.

It can sometimes be very surprising to find out how colleagues, friends and family view you. You will generally pick up clues about the impressions you make on others from the ways they behave towards you – although, of course, you may be wrong. Try asking a few different people how they view you. Their answers may also tell you something about *their* personality.

Clarification

People are said to lead happier lives if they are able to be aware of themselves and clear about the values that guide them. It is through this process that people are able to be open and honest when interacting with others. They understand their own motives. The development of this awareness should enable you to recognise when personal issues obstruct your ability to listen and respond to other people effectively (Peplau, 1988). Somebody who does not develop these skills (and you will come across people throughout your career who do not possess these skills) will allow their own insecurities and ideas to interfere with what they, or others, say or do. They are also likely to misinterpret what they see or hear (McLeod, 1998). Again, it is important to highlight that you can only remove the obstructions when you are able to recognise them in the first place.

Activity 2.9   *Reflection*

Identify a few core beliefs and values that you hold about nursing and make a note of them.

Consider and make a note of your answers to the following questions.

- Do I enjoy nursing?
- Why do I enjoy nursing?

continued overleaf . . .

---

continued . . .

- How do I benefit from being a nurse?
- Do I gain personally from nursing?

Now reflect upon your answers to those questions and make a note of all the personal gains you make through choosing a career as a nurse.

- Why do you think that it is vital for you to be aware of what you might gain personally from being in the role of a nurse?
- Do think that the value and belief that some people might hold about nurses being selfless people putting other people's happiness before their own is true?

There is no outline answer to this activity.

Earlier in the chapter there was some discussion about what might have brought you into a nursing career. Nurses may get satisfaction through seeing their patients recover from illnesses, especially when they know that they have made a difference to the recovery. Does this mean that nurses are really people who are selfishly getting their own needs met through helping people, in order feel better about themselves? Could this perhaps be true on some level? There are obvious risks involved because, as identified already, the nurse's personal needs may interfere if the nurse–patient relationship is the primary source for meeting those needs (Wosket, 2002). For example, relying on patients to satisfy the nurse's need for personal recognition, appreciation and validation is fraught with danger (Underman Boggs, 2007a). This will be discussed in more detail in Chapter 6 on communicating and relating. Nurses need to develop awareness of potential trouble spots, those personal needs that may interfere in their relationships with patients (Rogers, 1961).

Once you are able to draw on your past and present experiences and have some understanding of your own vulnerabilities and needs as a person, and as a nurse, you will be able to effectively work with your patients. That is not to say that you have to be totally aware of yourself – that is impossible; the aim is to be aware enough to enable you to make constructive use of your life experiences in order to enhance the helping relationships that you form with patients.

Chapter summary

When working with people it is important to be aware of how your own personal values and beliefs directly affect your interactions with patients. Your values and beliefs have the potential to restrict the development of effective relationships with patients. However, they can also play an integral role in enhancing your relationships should your value and belief systems be similar.

Effective relationships with your patients can be obstructed by personal values and beliefs due to the way they can function as perceptual filters. Perceptual filters allow some aspects of how a patient presents themselves both verbally and non-verbally to be accepted, while

continued . . .

others are rejected due to differing beliefs, which can manifest through opposing attitudes. This can have a negative effect on your listening skills.

Another way that personal values and beliefs can create problems in the relationship nurses have with their patients is through nurses imposing or projecting their own values and beliefs on to the patient. When values and beliefs are imposed on patients, they are often used (unconsciously) to judge patients. Whenever nurses make judgments about how patients 'should' or 'should not' be, feel or behave, there is a chance that they are evaluating patients in terms of their own value system. For this reason, you should always remember to reflect on these types of judgements.

Certain values and personal beliefs enhance and strengthen your ability to relate to patients. For example, a personal belief that all people at some level in relation to their capabilities are good, worthwhile and dependable can really work in favour of establishing an effective relationship with your patient. Such beliefs help create a climate of respect and regard for patients.

When relating to patients, nurses cannot be expected to abandon their values and personal beliefs. However, they need to be able to distinguish their own value and belief system from that of their patient. The more aware nurses are of their own values and personal beliefs, the less likely it is that interference will occur, and the more likely it is that the values that enhance effective relationships will be strengthened.

Activities: brief outline answers

Activity 2.2: Reflection (page 26)

- You may think that you now have increased responsibilities in view of yourself and others.
- You may feel you belong to a certain group of people and have some increased self-esteem linked to the high value people place on nurses.
- It is unlikely that your core values will have changed and it is unlikely that you have fundamentally changed. However, you may find that you have matured and are thinking more critically about your role in the world.
- Your core values and beliefs will be guiding you in what you do.

Activity 2.4: Critical thinking (page 28)

Jenny might have become overly involved with this patient through her own need to be liked. This means she would do anything to please the patient, which creates expectations from the patient that are unrealistic and not sustainable in the medium to long term. Professional boundaries have become blurred, leading to the problems experienced by Jenny. Jenny should accept that the patient does not want to speak to her and reapproach the patient when they are feeling able to talk. Jenny has not demonstrated any self-awareness in this situation.

Activity 2.7: Communication (page 33)

You may have experienced feelings of anger, guilt and frustration depending on how each person conducted themselves. The less intense the feelings, perhaps the more self-aware and appropriately you conducted your arguments in the interaction.

Further reading

Arnold, E and Underman Boggs, K (2011) *Interpersonal relationships: professional communication skills for nurses*, 6th edn. St Louis, MO: Saunders Elsevier.

This is a wonderful book if you would like something that is comprehensive about communicating and relating to others. It has some very helpful exercises to aid your learning.

McCabe, C and Timmins, F (2006) *Communication skills for nursing practice*. London: Palgrave Macmillan.

This book is specific to communication skills in nursing and is another comprehensive text that is very popular.

Neville, L (2009) *Interpersonal skills for the people professions: learning from practice*. London: Reflect Press.

This book is useful for all health and social care professionals and has a good skills-focused approach.

Useful websites

www.nursingplanet.com/pn/therapeutic_communication.html

This is a great open access nursing research and review site.

www.thecounsellorsguide.co.uk/

This site has lots of information that will build on the themes discussed within this chapter.

www.selfcreation.com/index.htm

This site has some great resources for aiding you in developing your self-awareness skills.

Chapter 3
The policy context for mental health care

Steven Trenoweth

NMC Standards for Pre-registration Nursing Education

This chapter will address the following competencies:

Domain 1: Professional values

1. All nurses must practise with confidence according to *The code: standards of conduct, performance and ethics for nurses and midwives* (NMC, 2008a), and within other recognised ethical and legal frameworks. They must be able to recognise and address ethical challenges relating to people's choices and decision-making about their care, and act within the law to help them and their families and carers find acceptable solutions.

2. All nurses must practise in a holistic, non-judgmental, caring and sensitive manner that avoids assumptions, supports social inclusion; recognises and respects individual choice; and acknowledges diversity. Where necessary, they must challenge inequality, discrimination and exclusion from access to care.

3. All nurses must support and promote the health, well-being, rights and dignity of people, groups, communities and populations. These include people whose lives are affected by ill health, disability, inability to engage, ageing or death. Nurses must act on their understanding of how these conditions influence public health.

4. All nurses must work in partnership with service users, carers, groups, communities and organisations. They must manage risk, and promote health and well-being while aiming to empower choices that promote self-care and safety.

5. All nurses must fully understand the nurse's various roles, responsibilities and functions, and adapt their practice to meet the changing needs of people, groups, communities and populations.

Domain 2: Communication and interpersonal skills

1. All nurses must build partnerships and therapeutic relationships through safe, effective and non-discriminatory communication. They must take account of individual differences, capabilities and needs.

Domain 3: Nursing practice and decision-making

5. All nurses must understand public health principles, priorities and practice in order to recognise and respond to the major causes and social determinants of health, illness and health inequalities. They must use a range of information and data to assess the

continued overleaf . . .

---

continued . . .

needs of people, groups, communities and populations, and work to improve health, well-being and experiences of healthcare; secure equal access to health screening, health promotion and healthcare; and promote social inclusion.

8. All nurses must provide educational support, facilitation skills and therapeutic nursing interventions to optimise health and well-being. They must promote self-care and management whenever possible, helping people to make choices about their healthcare needs, involving families and carers where appropriate, to maximise their ability to care for themselves.

9. All nurses must be able to recognise when a person is at risk and in need of extra support and protection and take reasonable steps to protect them from abuse.

Domain 4: Leadership, management and team working

1. All nurses must act as change agents and provide leadership through quality improvement and service development to enhance people's well-being and experiences of healthcare.

2. All nurses must systematically evaluate care and ensure that they and others use the findings to help improve people's experience and care outcomes and to shape future services.

3. All nurses must be able to identify priorities and manage time and resources effectively to ensure the quality of care is maintained or enhanced.

7. All nurses must work effectively across professional and agency boundaries, actively involving and respecting others' contributions to integrated person-centred care. They must know when and how to communicate with and refer to other professionals and agencies in order to respect the choices of service users and others, promoting shared decision making, to deliver positive outcomes and to coordinate smooth, effective transition within and between services and agencies.

NMC Essential Skills Clusters

Cluster: Care, compassion and communication

2. People can trust the newly registered graduate nurse to engage in person centred care empowering people to make choices about how their needs are met when they are unable to meet them for themselves.

4. People can trust a newly qualified graduate nurse to engage with them and their family or carers within their cultural environments in an acceptant and anti-discriminatory manner free from harassment and exploitation.

By the first progression point:

2. Respects people's rights.

3. Adopts a principled approach to care underpinned by the Code (NMC, 2008a).

continued overleaf . . .

continued . . .

Organisational aspects of care

9. People can trust the newly registered graduate nurse to treat them as partners and work with them to make a holistic and systematic assessment of their needs; to develop a personalised plan that is based on mutual understanding and respect for their individual situation promoting health and well-being, minimising risk of harm and promoting their safety at all times.

11. People can trust the newly registered graduate nurse to safeguard children and adults from vulnerable situations and support and protect them from harm.

Chapter aims

By the end of this chapter, you should be able to:

*   identify the mental health policy drivers for mental health care, including the stake-holder society and user involvement;
*   understand the economic and social costs of mental ill health;
*   identify key mental health policies, including those that aim to promote health, prevent suicide, care for carers and support vulnerable people.

Introduction

Look back at the case study about Sandra at the beginning of Chapter 1, on page 8. Sandra's case is not untypical. Many service users would like to feel more involved in their care and also more involved in their local communities, which being in paid work often facilitates. For people such as Sandra there is often no alternative but to receive state benefits, which may compound their feelings of disability and reinforce to the individual and society that the person is 'disabled' and in need of help and welfare. Sometimes people with mental health problems find it difficult to find work positions because of possible discrimination. Society has a responsibility to ensure social justice and fairness, and to ensure that all its citizens are able to actively participate in their communities (Repper and Perkins, 2009). There is, therefore, a need to ensure that policies are in place to support the person with mental health problems to regain their right of citizenship and to participate in all aspects of society.

Mental health care is a very political subject and is often the subject of much debate and policy development. At the heart of such debates are questions about: how and where mental health care should be provided; how it should be funded; what the role of mental health service users should be in policy and service development; and whether as a society we should spend our resources on treating mental disorders or promoting mental health. Historically, the care and treatment of people experiencing mental health problems have been located within specialist mental health services. However, as we can see from the NMC standards of competence, there is an expectation and professional requirement for nurses from whatever field to be able to respond to the holistic health care needs of their patients and service users. With regard to mental health care, this means that all nurses should have an understanding about mental ill health and understand the needs of, and provide quality care to, mental health service users wherever nursing care is required. It is therefore very important that you understand both context and policy background in mental health care. This will help you to appreciate why mental health services have been developed and how society seeks to respond to the needs of people who experience mental ill health.

In this chapter we consider some of the policy drivers for mental health care – past, present and future. These include: the economic and social costs of mental ill health; the rise of a 'stake-holding' society and user involvement movement; the promotion of holistic health and recovery; responding to vulnerability; the prevention of suicide; and the care and support of carers.

Activity 3.1   *Critical thinking*

Think for a moment about why there is a need for policies in mental health care. What policies do you think are needed to improve Sandra's participation in mental health care services and society overall?

An outline answer is given at the end of this chapter.

Mental health for all

Mental health is an issue for everyone in society. As we saw in Chapter 1, it is becoming increasingly clear that a purely medically based mental health treatment strategy is not sufficient to meet the complex care needs of the person experiencing mental distress. There have been calls for a more holistic approach that recognises psychological, social, emotional and spiritual as well as biological factors in mental health care (NIMHE, 2005b; Future Vision Coalition, 2009; Margereson and Trenoweth, 2010). For example, the Future Vision Coalition (a coalition of organisations including MIND, Centre for Mental Health, Rethink Mental Illness and the Mental Health Foundation among others) published a paper in 2009 calling for *A new vision for mental health*, which argued for a broader public health approach to mental health care, seeing that good mental health is important for everyone's overall good quality of life.

The Nursing and Midwifery Council (NMC) has reinforced the notion of holism in nursing care by stating, in its *Standards for pre-registration nursing education* (NMC, 2010a), that:

> *All nurses must practise in a holistic, non-judgmental, caring and sensitive manner that avoids assumptions, supports social inclusion; recognises and respects individual choice; and acknowledges diversity. Where necessary, they must challenge inequality, discrimination and exclusion from access to care.*
> (NMC, 2010a, p22)

In recent years, there has been a recognition that people with severe and enduring mental health problems have an increased vulnerability to a wide range of serious physical illnesses (Robson and Gray, 2007), such as coronary heart disease, diabetes and respiratory diseases (Mentality/ NIMHE, 2004). Additionally, they tend to have poorer access to medical care and are less likely to be offered routine health checks, such as blood pressure or cholesterol monitoring (DRC (Disability Rights Commission), 2006) or to receive health promotion advice (Mentality/ NIMHE, 2004). And of course as we saw in Chapter 2, people with physical health problems are also more vulnerable to mental ill health.

Recently, the policies *Choosing health: making healthy choices easier* (DH, 2004a) and *Choosing health: supporting the physical health needs of people with severe mental illness* (DH, 2006a) have sought to focus attention on developing programmes of health promotion for people with long-term and enduring mental health problems (Robson et al., 2008). The latter document in particular describes examples of good practice within mental health care services, for example, health improvement programmes, signposting people to health-promoting services (e.g. healthy walking groups, smoking cessation, dieting programmes), ensuring appropriate referral and access to various medical and other health care services.

However, it is true to say that while the physical health care of people with mental health problems has increased in importance on the policy agenda, there is still much work to be done to ensure equity of medical care compared with the general population (Phelan et al., 2001). Nurses have an important role here and can make a significant contribution to improve the physical well-being of people with mental health problems (DH, 2006b).

Activity 3.2 — *Reflection*

Think for a moment about how you as a nurse can contribute to the mental health care of your patients and service users. What skills, knowledge, values and attitudes will you need to have in order to respond to the holistic care needs of those in need of your nursing care?

An outline answer is given at the end of the chapter.

Economic and social costs

An important influence on policy development is the economic and social cost of mental ill health. It is currently estimated that the cost of mental ill health to the UK economy in 2009–10 was £105.2 billion. This includes direct costs, such as those involved in the direct provision of care – for 2008–09 this was £10.4 billion or 11 per cent of all gross NHS expenditure (DH, 2010) – but also other costs associated with reduction in economic output and impact on quality of life (Centre for Mental Health, 2010).

In recent years, there have been other policy developments that have had a direct impact on the lives of people with mental health problems, particularly those with long-term conditions. In recent years, for example, UK governments have had stated policies of reducing perceived dependence on welfare benefits, with an aspiration of 80 per cent employment. For example, the New Labour government's policies (such as 'Welfare to Work', 'New Deal' and 'Flexible New Deal') sought to support skills development and encourage people to work, recognising that a lack of employment seems to lead to multiple social and economic disadvantage. More recently, the UK government has announced policies of welfare reform as a way of reducing the budget deficit.

Encouraging people to return to work after experiencing mental health problems has many more advantages than just economics. Being in paid work is an important part of our lives. In employment, there is a greater potential for social contacts and activities that offer a sense of fulfilment and achievement. We may argue that is quite right that there should be policies that assist in supporting people who are able to return to work. For people with mental health problems, being in paid employment can assist their inclusion into local communities and promote a sense of citizenship. Many people with mental health problems wish to work (ODPM (Office of the Deputy Prime Minister), 2004) but one-third are unemployed or economically inactive and almost three-quarters of those with a diagnosis of schizophrenia are out of work (ONS, 2002). Indeed, for people with long-term mental ill health, finding and securing work can be particularly problematic (Future Vision Coalition, 2009), perhaps due, in part, to the increased likelihood that people with ongoing mental health problems are more likely to have left school at 16 and with no qualifications (ONS, 2002).

There is also evidence that people with existing serious and enduring mental health problems are stigmatised and discriminated against (DH, 1999a; ODPM, 2004; Future Vision Coalition, 2009) despite the Disability Discrimination Act (1995), which makes discrimination against disabled people an offence. Media representations of mental disorders can reinforce stereotypes of individuals with mental health problems in society (Kemp, 2008). The effect of such stigmas is that people often find that they are socially excluded from communities (Future Vision Coalition, 2009). Such exclusion may also, in turn, contribute to the development and maintenance of mental ill health and to possible relapse among those with existing problems (Jenkins et al., 2008) and thus represents a vicious circle in terms of difficulties they may experience with engagement and participation in communities (ODPM, 2004). As such, the individual's search for employment (or their return to work after experiencing mental ill health) is an important part of mental health policy (DH, 2001b). This not only helps people to claim their rights of citizenship but also makes a potentially significant contribution to the maintenance of good mental health and is supportive of recovery. Such policies apply not only to the mental health care system but also to the wider world of work.

People with mental health problems often experience other forms of social disadvantage. In addition to their possible exclusion from communities, and a severe perceived lack of social support, they are more likely to have financial problems and be single, divorced or separated; and they are far more likely to be living in cramped rented accommodation than the general population (ONS, 2002). This places an additional burden on vulnerable people who may be recovering from, or living with, mental health issues and is likely to have a detrimental effect on their health, well-being and overall quality of life. There is, therefore, a requirement placed upon health and social care services to offer practical support in relation to dealing with financial, accommodation and relationship difficulties.

In 2011, the government launched its new mental health strategy for England *No health without mental health* (DH, 2011a). This strategy recognises the economic, social and personal cost of mental ill health and proposes a number of key developments to improve the mental health of people with existing mental health problems, while seeking to prevent mental ill health where this is possible. The strategy also recognises the social inequalities (such as those described above – lack of access to work, poor housing, isolation from communities and so forth) that people with mental ill health may experience and how this contributes to further mental distress. The government argues that the strategy is *both a public mental health strategy and a strategy for social justice* (DH, 2011a, p3).

Key mental health policies

It is not possible in this chapter to cover all policies that impact on mental health care. However, in the following pages we have sought to highlight the key policy documents and approaches that have influenced contemporary mental health care, so that you will be able to understand how society seeks to support people such as Sandra. In particular, we will examine: the importance of service user involvement; promoting mental health and recovery; holism; how mental health services seek to support and care for vulnerable people by the Care Programme Approach (CPA); suicide prevention; and caring about carers.

Over the last two decades in particular there have been a number of significant policies that have changed the way in which mental health services deliver care (Kemp, 2008). The New Labour government's election in 1997 placed emphasis on citizenship, the importance of the individual's participation in society and the idea of a 'stakeholding' society in which everyone participated.

A central point for the New Labour government's approach to mental health care was the National Service Framework for Mental Health (NSFMH) (DH, 1999b), which, for example, set out to modernise mental health care by establishing a set of national quality standards. Such standards involved: protection to the public and effective care to those with perceived mental health needs; increased access to a full range of services; reduced suicide rates; and support for the carers and families of people with mental health problems.

The NSFMH (DH, 1999b) policy also influenced service development and increased the range of community-based services supporting people at a time of crisis as an alternative to hospital admissions. These included:

- Early Intervention in Psychosis (EIPS) (for those under 35 years and in need of early and intensive support) (DH, 1999b, 2001);
- Assertive Outreach (intensive support aimed at managing care in the community for people with serious mental illness who are difficult to engage with an explicit aim of reducing hospital admissions) (DH, 1999b, 2001);
- Crisis Resolution and Home Treatment (CRHT) Teams (often 24-hour services offering intensive support for acute problems) (DH, 2001b; CSIP, 2006).

Some mental health services also provide specialist services for local communities, such as black and ethnic minorities, mentally disordered offenders, children and adolescents, people with substance use issues and people with mental health problems who are homeless (DH, 2001b).

User involvement

In 1997, the New Labour government published its strategy for the health service, *The new NHS: modern, dependable* (DH, 1997), which stated: *The Government will take special steps to ensure that the experience of users and carers is central to the work of the NHS* (DH, 1997, p66).

Since this time, 'user involvement' has indeed become an increasingly important central point of many policy initiatives (Hewitt, 2005), and there is an expectation and requirement that service users will be involved in all aspects of their care and will be able to influence service provision by full and active consultation. Charities and voluntary organisations (such as Rethink Mental Illness, MIND and so forth) have been vital in representing the views of service users, ensuring that such views influence policy development at local and governmental level.

According to Kemp (2008), there are both 'top-down' policy pressures to involve service users and 'bottom-up' demands from service users for increasing their involvement in all aspects of the mental health system, such as: advocacy; direct provision of care; service monitoring; user-led research; and the training and education of professional staff. At the level of care delivery, service users themselves now expect to be involved in decisions about treatment, and there is a require-ment for nurses to provide care that is user-sensitive and based on what users themselves feel are most helpful to them in their recovery (DH, 1999b, 2006b; Rose 2001). Indeed, this has found expression in the government's White Paper *Liberating the NHS*, which states: *no decision about me without me* (DH, 2010, p3). Mental health charities and voluntary organisations have led the way here and have been instrumental in policy formulation and for campaigning to ensure that the voice of service users is heard. The profile of Rethink Mental Illness below illustrates how central user involvement is to their work.

Profile of a voluntary organisation and mental health charity: Rethink Mental Illness

Rethink Mental Illness, the leading national mental health membership charity, works to help everyone affected by severe mental illness recover a better quality of life. It provides hope and empowerment through effective services and support to all those in need of help, and campaigns for change through greater awareness and understanding.

Providing practical support
Rethink Mental Illness runs over 135 groups, which meet regularly to provide carers and people with severe mental illness with a support network in their local area.

Providing services
Rethink Mental Illness is the largest national voluntary sector provider of mental health services with 338 services. Services include crisis services, services within the criminal justice system, advocacy, carer and community support, psychological therapies, employment and training, practical help and advice services, supported housing, nursing and residential care, and services dedicated to black and minority ethnic communities.

Campaigning

Rethink Mental Illness is dedicated to creating a world where prejudice and discrimination against people who experience mental health problems are eliminated and everyone affected by severe mental illness gets first-class treatment and care. Over its 30-year history it has successfully campaigned for changes to major pieces of legislation and government policy on key issues such as health and social care and benefits. In consultation with its members, it has developed policies that have influenced the modernisation of mental health services.

Changing attitudes

Rethink Mental Illness has piloted innovative approaches to changing society's attitudes to mental illness and now it is implementing them on a national level as part of Time to Change, England's most ambitious programme to end discrimination faced by people who experience mental illness. Rethink Mental Illness trains people to speak about real experiences in the media so that the public get the real story about severe mental illness and it encourages people in high-profile positions to talk about their experiences of mental illness. It challenges journalists' misconceptions of conditions such as schizophrenia with facts and real-life examples.

Changing practice

Rethink Mental Illness offers education and training to key groups of people that have the power to change the lives of people affected by severe mental illness. It has trained thousands of medical students, teachers, police and school children. All the training is needs-led and designed and delivered by mental health professionals, alongside people with real experience of severe mental illness and caring.

Research

Rethink Mental Illness's research team looks at the real experiences of people affected by severe mental illness to strengthen the evidence base on what works and what does not work in mental health. It works with people who use their services, staff and members to develop research plans. It works in partnership with universities, hospitals and other charities to contribute to best practice in mental health and uses their research findings as the basis for campaigns to shape government policy.

Reproduced by permission of Rethink Mental Illness (www.rethink.org)

Kemp (2008) has argued that the development of service user involvement in mental health care has taken place in the context of other changes in society, such as the empowerment of individuals, which reflect individual human rights and the rise of a more consumer-focused health services (Griffiths, 1983). Perhaps the clearest expression of this in recent years has been the UK government's White Paper *Liberating the NHS* (DH, 2010). This approach seeks to ensure that the NHS is more accountable to patients, and that the patient is central to care. This will, it is posed, ensure that the patient is in charge of making decisions about their care, including choosing what treatment and which provider will best meet their health care needs, based on access information about the best health care services.

Promoting health and recovery

Another very important policy approach in mental health care is that of the promotion of health and recovery. The National Service Framework for Mental Health (DH, 1999b) required that *health and social services should promote mental health for all, working with individuals and communities, whilst combating discrimination against individuals and groups with mental health problems and promoting their social inclusion.* Important to the promotion of health and recovery is a focus on a hopeful, optimistic, positive approach to mental health care (DH, 2001b), where people who have experienced or are experiencing mental ill health are supported to live a meaningful life of personal value and worth (NIMHE, 2005b; Jenkins et al., 2008). You can read more about this in Chapter 2. In recent years, this has found expression in mental health care policies that have emphasised:

- the importance of working in partnership within the context of a supportive and empathic professional nursing relationship;
- shared decision making between mental health service users and nurses;
- nursing care that reflects the service user's preference based on informed discussions;
- a recognition that individuals have personal strengths and assets as well as problems and needs;
- support to deal with the future and cope with challenges that mental health problems may bring (Future Vision Coalition, 2009).

Such approaches have been emphasised by the *Chief Nursing Officer's review of mental health nursing* (DH, 2006b) and have also formed the basis of the Labour government's *New horizons: a shared vision for mental health* (DH, 2009) policy framework. For the National Institute for Mental Health for England (NIMHE) recovery is:

> *what people experience themselves as they become empowered to manage their lives in a manner that allows them to achieve a fulfilling, meaningful life and a contributing sense of belonging in their communities.*
> (NIMHE, 2005b, p2)

As such, recovery approaches have emphasised the need to assist people to develop personal resources and strategies embedded within a context of developing wider, informal social supports. This represents a movement away from the emphasis on 'technical' and medical interventions (Faulkner and Layzell, 2000), which have historically been the focus of mental health care. In keeping with the notion of citizenship and the development of a 'stakeholding' society, the new recovery approaches stress the importance of developing meaningful professional alliances and relationships between nurses and service users with a focus on enabling, facilitating and supporting individuals on their journeys to recovery.

Caring for vulnerable people

The Care Programme Approach (CPA) policy was introduced in 1990 by the then Conservative government, and has been central to government policy since that time (DH, 2008). CPA aimed to ensure that vulnerable people with mental health problems who have been in contact with mental health services receive the ongoing care they need. The policy aimed to provide:

- systematic arrangements for assessing the health and social needs of people accepted into specialist mental health services;
- the development of a care plan that identified the health and social care, documenting not only agreed mental health care and treatment but also plans to secure employment, occupational activity, accommodation and adequate housing, and entitlement to benefits;
- the appointment of a key worker (care co-ordinator) to keep in close touch with the service user, and to monitor and co-ordinate care; and
- regular review and, where necessary, agreed changes to the care plan.

The implementation of CPA arrangements, while embedded in mental health care service provision, has not been straightforward, and it has been poorly implemented with poor service user involvement being reported (Rose, 2001; Social Services Inspectorate, 2002; Healthcare Commission, 2005). Furthermore, some service users have been unclear what CPA is for. Such problems can significantly undermine the effectiveness of any care plan and the experience of mental health services.

Revised procedures were introduced in 1999 (DH, 1999b) and embedded into the NSFMH's (DH, 1999b) Standard 4, which required that all mental health service users in need of CPA should:

- receive care that optimises engagement, anticipates or prevents a crisis, and reduces risk;
- have a copy of their care plan, which should include the action to be taken in a crisis by the service user, their carer and their care co-ordinator, and advise their GP how they should respond if the service user needs additional help and is regularly reviewed by their care co-ordinator;
- be able to access services 24 hours a day, 365 days a year.

In 2008, a further refocusing of the CPA policy was undertaken in the New Labour government's Refocusing the Care Programme Approach (DH, 2008). The policy sought to re-emphasise the personalisation of mental health care and that active service user involvement and engagement must be at the heart of the approach, along with reducing distress and promoting social inclusion and recovery.

Preventing suicide

The NSFMH (DH, 1999b) sought to reduce the number of suicides by 2010 by one-fifth to 7.3 per 100,000 (DH, 1999b, 2001b, 2002). Recognising that suicide prevention requires a health and social care community approach, the policy sought to reduce suicide rates by:

- promoting mental health for all, working with individuals and communities;
- increasing mental health care and support in primary care;
- ensuring that anyone with a mental health problem can contact local services via the primary care team, a helpline or a casualty department;
- ensuring that individuals with severe and enduring mental health problems have a CPA care plan that meets their specific needs, including access to services round the clock;

- providing safe hospital accommodation for individuals who need it;
- enabling individuals caring for someone with severe mental health problems to receive the support that they need to continue to care.

In 2002 the Department for Health published the *National suicide prevention strategy for England* (DH, 2002), which built on the NSFMH by seeking to: reduce the suicide risk in high-risk groups; promote well-being in the wider community; and reduce lethality and availability of suicide methods, for example, by reducing the pack size of non-prescription paracetamol (DH, 2002). The latest statistics (ONS, 2011) continue to show a downward trend until 2008 but have recently shown a slight increase. In 2007 there were 5,377 suicides in adults aged 15 and over – 940 less than in 1991 (6,317). In 2009, there were 5,675 suicides. The suicide rate in 2009 for men was 17.5 per 100,000 population, and for women was 5.2 per 100,000 population (ONS, 2011).

Caring about carers

Many people with ongoing mental health problems live with their family or with friends (DH, 1999b; Jenkins et al., 2008). Unfortunately, the needs of carers have often been overlooked. While many carers often undertake caring willingly and may find their role rewarding, the strains and responsibilities can take its toll, both financially and emotionally. Carers, for example, are twice as likely to have mental health problems themselves if they provide substantial care (DH, 1999b, 2001; ODPM, 2004). In recent years, it is recognised that in order to fulfil such an important role, carers themselves may require support from health and social care services. This may involve not only practical help and assistance regarding benefit entitlements, but also information about the care and treatment options available to their friend or relative and what to do, and who to contact, should a crisis arise (DH, 1999b). Standard 6 of the NSFMH (DH, 1999b) requires that all individuals who provide extensive care for a person who is subject to CPA arrangements should:

- have an assessment of their caring, physical and mental health needs repeated on at least an annual basis;
- have their own written care plan, which is given to them and implemented in discussion with them.

Mental health services are therefore required to ensure that carers are offered the necessary support to assist them to meet their own emotional, financial, social, mental and physical needs.

Activity 3.3   *Critical thinking*

Outline the strengths and limitations of the policies and strategies described above when considering care for people with mental health issues. Is there anything you believe that has been omitted from such policies?

An outline answer is given at the end of the chapter.

Chapter summary

In this chapter, we have examined a number of policies that have sought to respond to the needs of people with mental health problems, many of whom are subject to stigma and social exclusion from communities and work. Policies have placed an emphasis on public involvement, citizenship and on the importance of the individual's participation in society and the idea of an empowered 'stakeholding' society based on social participation. Key mental health policies in recent years have focused on: the importance of service user involvement; promoting mental health and recovery; holism; the Care Programme Approach (CPA); suicide prevention; and caring about carers.

More recently mental health nursing policy (DH, 2006b) has placed an emphasis on assisting the whole person on the road to recovery, and this requires nurses to deliver comprehensive and holistic care, from clinically effective medical interventions to improving meaningful employment prospects, improving diet and physical health, improving social support and satisfying personal relationships. However, the NMC's *Standards for pre-registration nursing education* (NMC, 2010a) emphasise the importance of holistic care across all fields and that while mental health nurses may specialise in such care, the delivery of mental health care is a responsibility of all nurses.

The recent White Paper *Liberating the NHS* (DH, 2010) will be the blueprint for mental health care in the immediate years to come. Its policy approach, with an emphasis on the centrality of the service user choice and experience, and empowered health care staff delivering outcome-focused care, will open a new era of mental health care.

Activities: brief outline answers

Activity 3.1: Critical thinking (page 41)

Policies are often needed to direct service provision and to ensure that there is a consistency of approach. In this sense, policies are useful to guide the development of strategies. Policies can also be the benchmark against which services can be assessed and held accountable. When there are finite resources, policies are useful for ensuring that specific objectives are achieved. As we shall see from Chapter 5, in addition to policies there are also legal requirements to support the rights and citizenship of people with mental health problems.

With regard to Sandra you might have said that there needs to be policies that ensure her right of choice in care and treatment and support her efforts to return to work. You might also have said that there should be polices that seek to help her to maintain and improve her own holistic well-being while ensuring that at times of vulnerability support is available for her and those who may care for her

Activity 3.2: Reflection (page 42)

In answering this question you may wish to consult the standards of competence for your particular field. This can be found in the NMC's *Standards for pre-registration nursing education* (NMC, 2010a), available at: **http://standards.nmc-uk.org/PreRegNursing/statutory/competencies/Pages/Competencies.aspx**

It is likely that you have listed your skills, knowledge, attitudes and values under the following domains.

1. Professional values.
2. Communication and interpersonal skills.
3. Nursing practice and decision-making.
4. Leadership, management and team working.

For example, if you are an adult nursing student you might have said that you might need to ensure that you are mindful of the mental distress experienced by your patients; that you would listen to their issues in a sensitive and non-judgemental way; that you would attempt to build trust; that you would communicate in a clear, jargon-free way; that you would promote choice; and that you would advocate for your patients, ensuring that the nursing team you worked with are as mindful of the mental health needs of your patients as you are.

Activity 3.3: Critical thinking (page 49)

The overall purpose of policies and strategies is to ensure that there is consistency across communities in terms of the sort of care and treatment that should be available for people who experience mental ill health. Strategies such as *No health without mental health* (DH, 2011a) seek to address health improvement with a much wider strategy for social justice and of reducing social inequality. We may argue that such approaches should be at governmental level to ensure that sufficient resources are available, and that all people, regardless of where they live, will benefit. However, policies that seek to ensure national coverage may not be responsive to the specific needs of individuals or particular communities. For example, some communities may experience more disadvantage than others due to factors such as poor quality housing, greater rates of poverty and exposure to crime. Such factors may be more prevalent in inner city areas than rural communities. However, we might argue that in the latter there is less access to rewarding and meaningful work. Policies are not likely, in any case, to be responsive to the needs of all people at all times so it is inevitable that some individuals may find that polices and strategies do not always accommodate their specific needs.

Further reading

Reynolds, J, Muston, R, Heller, T, Leach, J, McCormick, M, Wallcraft, J and Walsh, M (eds) (2009) *Mental health still matters.* London: Palgrave.

A collection of readings and essays that explores the current context of mental health care services and policy within the UK. Section 2 in particular examines the issue of citizenship and inclusivity.

Useful websites

www.rethink.org/

The main website for Rethink Mental Illness. This site gives an excellent overview of their work and how they contribute to and influence policy development within the UK. It is also an excellent resource and contains much useful information for nurses of all fields to develop their knowledge and understanding of contemporary mental health care.

www.dh.gov.uk/en/Healthcare/Mentalhealth/index.htm

The Department of Health's main pages for mental health with news and information on policy, consultations and policy development.

Chapter 4
Mental and physical health care needs

Steven Trenoweth

NMC Standards for Pre-registration Nursing Education

This chapter will address the following competencies:

Domain 1: Professional values

5. All nurses must fully understand the nurse's various roles, responsibilities and functions, and adapt their practice to meet the changing needs of people, groups, communities and populations.

Domain 2: Communication and interpersonal skills

4. All nurses must recognise when people are anxious or in distress and respond effectively, using therapeutic principles, to promote their well-being, manage personal safety and resolve conflict. They must use effective communication strategies and negotiation techniques to achieve best outcomes, respecting the dignity and human rights of all concerned. They must know when to consult a third party and how to make referrals for advocacy, mediation or arbitration.

Domain 3: Nursing practice and decision-making

2. All nurses must possess a broad knowledge of the structure and functions of the human body, and other relevant knowledge from the life, behavioural and social sciences as applied to health, ill health, disability, ageing and death. They must have an in-depth knowledge of common physical and mental health problems and treatments in their own field of practice, including co-morbidity and physiological and psychological vulnerability.

3. All nurses must carry out comprehensive, systematic nursing assessments that take account of relevant physical, social, cultural, psychological, spiritual, genetic and environmental factors, in partnership with service users and others through interaction, observation and measurement.

4. All nurses must ascertain and respond to the physical, social and psychological needs of people, groups and communities. They must then plan, deliver and evaluate safe, competent, person-centred care in partnership with them, paying special attention to changing health needs during different life stages, including progressive illness and death, loss and bereavement.

continued overleaf . . .

continued . . .

7. All nurses must be able to recognise and interpret signs of normal and deteriorating mental and physical health and respond promptly to maintain or improve the health and comfort of the service user, acting to keep them and others safe.

Domain 4: Leadership, management and team working

4. All nurses must be self-aware and recognise how their own values, principles and assumptions may affect their practice. They must maintain their own personal and professional development, learning from experience, through supervision, feedback, reflection and evaluation.

NMC Essential Skills Clusters

Cluster: Organisational aspects of care

9. People can trust the newly registered graduate nurse to treat them as partners and work with them to make a holistic and systematic assessment of their needs; to develop a personalised plan that is based on mutual understanding and respect for their individual situation promoting health and well-being, minimising risk of harm and promoting their safety at all times.

By the second progression point:

9. Undertakes the assessment of physical, emotional, psychological, social, cultural and spiritual needs, including risk factors by working with the person and records, shares and responds to clear indicators and signs.

By entry to the register:

12. In partnership with the person, their carers and their families, makes a holistic, person centred and systematic assessment of physical, emotional, psychological, social, cultural and spiritual needs, including risk, and together develops a comprehensive personalised plan of nursing care.

Chapter aims

By the end of this chapter, you should be able to:

* understand the potential links between mental and physical ill health;
* understand and describe the risk factors for physical ill health among people experiencing mental health problems;
* discuss the holistic role of all nurses in providing care to people with healthcare needs.

Introduction

There is much evidence that people who experience mental ill health do not enjoy good physical health when compared to the general population. It is also true to say that people who experience poor physical health, such as those with chronic, long-term conditions, likewise do not always enjoy good mental health. As such, the ability of nurses to deliver holistic care is an important feature of modern nursing practice. In this chapter, we explore the potential links between mental and physical ill health, and explore the risk factors for physical ill health among people experiencing mental health problems. Finally, we look at the holistic role of all nurses in providing care to people with health care needs.

Mental health of people with physical health problems

Activity 4.1   *Critical thinking*

Think for a moment and make notes on why someone with a physical illness might experience poor mental health. Revisit Swinton's (2001) model on page 19 in Chapter 1 – how might a person who is ill feel *holistically*? That is, how might this disease affect our social, physical, psychological, emotional and spiritual dimensions of self?

An outline answer is given at the end of the chapter.

Theory summary: Swinton's holistic model of health (Swinton, 2001)

A holistic model has five inter-connected dimensions.

- Physical (the biological aspect of our selves).
- Social (our relationships with others).
- Emotional (the way in which we feel about ourselves and our lives).
- Psychological (beliefs and perceptions that we hold about ourselves and others).
- Spiritual (the meaning that we attach to our lives).

As nurses we care for people in a variety of situations and contexts. We will often see people who have **co-morbid mental distress** (that is, mental distress that exists at the same time as other health issues), and this may have an effect on the way both health issues develop. People with physical illnesses have comparatively high rates of mental health problems, and there is evidence that among people with various physical illnesses their psychological distress goes unacknowledged and often is not recognised. Those who are depressed tend to experience pain more, which has an impact on both the trajectory of and the recovery from illness (Gureje, 2007). Without such recognition the person in distress may not receive the help they need to support them at difficult times in their lives. The key message here is that in order to understand the mental distress a person might be experiencing, we must look to the whole person.

'Good' mental health, we may argue, can only result if each dimension of Swinton's holistic model (see Theory summary box) is in harmony. That is, when we experience good mental health, we may feel physically fit and able; we may feel that we make a valid and worthwhile contribution to the lives of others; we may feel positive about ourselves and our lives; we hold ourselves in esteem and as a person of worth; and we feel our lives have direction, purpose and meaning. However, this would seem to imply that people with chronic or long-term conditions cannot have good mental health, which is clearly not the case. However, painful, debilitating and disabling health problems are more likely to undermine our subjective experiences of good mental health and hence may lead to mental distress.

Look again at the case study about John on page 20 in Chapter 1 which suggests that John has experienced a severe asthma attack and that his quietness and uncommunicativeness are related to his fears over his physical health. His lack of personal hygiene may be construed as stemming from problems with mobility due to possible breathing problems. There may be a suspicion of an underlying chest infection that has exacerbated his asthma. However, as we shall see in this chapter, John's physical health and apparent mental ill health may combine to affect the prognosis of both his respiratory problems and mood. This is because there are strong links between physical and mental ill health.

In extreme cases, people who experience serious, chronic, painful physical illnesses are at heightened risk of suicide. In a recent study of people who committed suicide in the south of England who contacted NHS Direct prior to ending their lives, over 50 per cent reported physical problems while 30 per cent reported mental health problems (Bessant et al., 2008). Links between mental and physical ill health are often 'bi-directional'. That is, a person's physical health may influence mental health ill health and vice versa. This appears to be particularly true for the experience of pain. Chronic pain, it appears, contributes to a higher incidence of depression, but depression also seems to affect our experience of pain (Gureje, 2007). Likewise, peace of mind appears to offer relief from pain, while fear and anger appear to amplify pain (Bope et al., 2004). Most of us can think of examples from our own experience, at work or otherwise, that support these research findings. Among people with physical health problems emotional problems are not uncommon, especially if those health issues are chronic (NICE, 2009c). For example, there is an increased risk of depression among people with heart failure, diabetes, strokes, chronic obstructive pulmonary disease (COPD), Parkinson's disease, multiple sclerosis and end-stage renal failure (Hackett et al., 2005). People with asthma also have higher rates of both depression and anxiety (Lavoie et al., 2006). The Royal College of Physicians and Royal College of Psychiatrists have estimated that approximately 15 per cent of medical hospital in-patients may experience anxiety and depression (RCP, 1995). In some circumstances, such difficulties can lead to a person experiencing concurrent mental ill health to such an extent that mental health care and psychiatric interventions may be needed. Such mental health problems can, in turn, affect their prognosis and recovery or lead to an exacerbation of the physical health problem.

Having a mental health problem that co-exists with a physical health problem can seriously affect both the person's ability to cope with their physical health problems and their quality of life. Take, for example, the condition of diabetes. Symptoms of depression such as low motivation, reduced energy levels and reduced appetite can lead to poor glycaemic control as the person may feel less able to prepare and eat a healthy diet. This can, in turn, increase the risk of complications associated with diabetes (affecting the eyes, nerves, kidneys and feet, for example), which can, in turn, exacerbate symptoms of depression. So, for a person with diabetes, depression can lead to a downward spiral, in which the symptoms of diabetes are less well managed, leading to an increased risk of complications, which can lead to a worsening of the symptoms of depression (Ciechanowski et al., 2000). As such, it is important to realise that care and treatment of the mental health problems of a physically unwell person can also be very beneficial in terms of improving their prognosis and overall quality of life. In diabetes, for example, there is evidence that active treatment of depression can improve and regulate glycaemic control (Goldney et al., 2004).

Sometimes a physical health problem can appear to be a mental health problem. For example, 'delirium' (acute confusional state) often has a rapid onset and is a condition characterised by changeable levels of consciousness and confusion with an impaired ability to think and concentrate; it is thought to affect 30 per cent of older people admitted to medical areas (McManus et al., 2007). Delirium often results from infections, malnutrition, lack of sleep and water, fever, brain injury, drug withdrawal or intoxication and can lead to hyperactivity (increased energy and activity) or hypoactivity (such as lethargy and reduced activity). Here, it is very important for the nurse to recognise when apparent symptoms of mental ill health might be an indication of an underlying physical illness and to be mindful of the greater risk that this might pose for the ill person in terms of their personal safety, especially when the person may have dementia or be physically frail.

Physical health of people with mental health problems

There is evidence that people with mental health problems have poorer access to, and receipt of, medical care than the general population (including less frequent hospitalisation for medical care), and as a consequence this group tends to have poorer physical health and higher mortality rates (DRC, 2006). Mentality/NIMHE (2004) estimated that a person diagnosed with schizophrenia can expect to live ten years fewer than the general population. However, having a mental health issue can itself lead to an increased risk of developing physical health problems. For example, people with mental health problems have increased risks of developing diabetes (Gough and Peveler, 2004), and those with depression are twice as likely to have heart problems a year following their diagnosis (Carney et al., 1988).

Activity 4.2   *Evidence-based practice and research*

Make some notes on why you feel someone with a mental health problem might not enjoy the same levels of physical health as the general population.

An outline answer is given at the end of this chapter.

In 2006, the Disability Rights Commission (DRC, 2006) investigated the apparent health care inequalities experienced by people with mental health problems and those with learning disabilities. The findings were shocking. The investigation found that people with schizophrenia, bipolar disorder and depression are more likely to have diabetes, coronary heart disease, respiratory problems (such as COPD) and hypertension. There is an increased risk of cancers, such as breast and bowel cancers, which tend to occur at a younger age and with a poorer survival rate than the general population. This was echoed by Harris and Barraclough (1998) who reviewed 152 studies and found that mental ill health was associated with an increased risk of premature death.

More recently, attention has been drawn to the sexual health of people with mental health problems, particularly among younger people in this group (Sheild et al., 2005), who appear to be at heightened risk of contracting sexually transmitted infections. Schoolchildren with mental health problems are twice as likely as their peers to be sexually active and to engage in unsafe sexual practices. Teenage girls with mental health problems are more likely to become pregnant (Kessler et al., 1997). Conversely, it appears that young women with a diagnosis of schizophrenia have lower rates of fertility from their mid-twenties (Howard et al., 2002), possibly due to the effects of medication use (see below).

It is very clear that all nurses have a duty and responsibility to identify physical ill health among people with mental health problems. There is, however, much evidence of poor detection of physical illness among people with serious mental health problems. Sometimes this may be due to a lack of willingness of mental health service users to engage with health services or to accept and act on health education advice. However, there is evidence that this also seems related to the ability and willingness of health care professionals to engage with people with mental health problems. On occasions there may be an over-emphasis on mental health issues, which has meant that the physical health care needs of an individual is overlooked (Dean et al., 2001; Friedli and Dardis, 2002). Worse, reported physical symptoms may be dismissed and seen to be connected to the mental ill health and 'all in the person's mind' (Seymour, 2003). There is also an inaccurate assumption that people with mental health problems do not care about their physical health (Mentality/NIMHE, 2004). However, as Seymour (2003) found, mental health service users are, in fact, concerned about their physical health and value, and welcome health promotion information and advice. Nurses must therefore reflect upon and challenge their assumptions about the overall health care needs of this client group.

Risk factors for physical ill health among those with mental health problems

Nurses must be mindful of the increased risk of physical illness and disease among a mental health client group. There should be early interventions when a risk is identified to slow the disease progression or to reduce the possibility of complications from physical ill health. Nurses must proactively assess those factors that increase such risk and wherever possible proactively work with individuals to promote health.

Identifying risk factors for any physical illness is a complex process. It is likely that several 'lifestyle' factors (such as smoking, poor diet and a lack of exercise) may combine to cumulatively impact on the physical health of people with mental health problems. This has implications for both quality of life and mortality rates for such groups. McCreadie (2003) found that people diagnosed with schizophrenia were exposed to more risk in terms of lifestyle factors compared to the poorest socio-economic group within the general population. It is vital, therefore, that you understand the range of risk factors to which an individual may be exposed so that you can develop effective nursing and health-promotion strategies. In this section, therefore, we will look at the main lifestyle and risk factors that may affect the physical health of people with mental health problems.

Smoking

Evidence seems to indicate that people with mental health problems tend to smoke at higher rates, and at higher levels (that is, smoking over 20 cigarettes per day) than the general population (Brown et al., 1999; McCloughen, 2003). For example, Kelly and McCreadie (1999) found that nearly 70 per cent of people diagnosed with schizophrenia were heavy smokers compared with approximately 10 per cent in the general population.

Activity 4.3   *Critical thinking*

Why, in general, do people smoke? Are there any additional reasons why someone experiencing mental distress might smoke?

An outline answer is given at the end of this chapter.

There have been many reasons put forward to explain the higher incidences of smoking among people experiencing mental ill health. McCloughen (2003) suggested that nicotine might act to alleviate some of the symptoms of mental health problems and the side effects of medication. For example, nicotine is a stimulant and has a potential energising effect when one is feeling tired and lethargic. Conversely, smoking can, for some, be relaxing. However, we must remember that people who smoke often do so because of a physiological addiction, for social reasons and for pleasure, and because it is a habitual part of their daily routine (Robson and Gray, 2005). In this regard, factors among this client group that maintain a smoking habit are the same as the general population. There is also some evidence that smoking is considered to be a part of the mental health culture. Stubbs and Gardner (2004), for example, found that over half of people who worked in mental health care settings felt that smoking was helpful in terms of developing a therapeutic relationship. That is, smoking was felt to be a useful mechanism between the nurse and service user to forge a social connection. Nurses who smoke may not place an emphasis on smoking cessation, increasing the risk of physical ill health and premature death among this client group – which is clearly incompatible with the health-promoting role of a nurse.

Diet

A good diet is an important protective factor contributing to good physical health.

Activity 4.4   *Critical thinking*

What is a 'good' diet? Make some notes on what you feel are the main criteria for a healthy diet.

An outline answer is given at the end of this chapter.

A poor diet increases the risk of some forms of cancer (such as bowel cancer), diabetes, cardio-vascular disease and hypertension, and it is clear that people with mental health problems have a poorer diet than the general population (Brown et al., 1999; McCreadie, 2003). Brown et al. (1999) assessed the diets of 102 people diagnosed with schizophrenia, finding an intake of higher rates of saturated fat. None of the group studied was eating the recommended weekly minimum of five portions of fruit or vegetables each day and one portion of oily fish (FSA (Food Standards Agency), 2001). This may account for the finding by McCreadie (2003) that among a sample of people diagnosed with schizophrenia, over 50 per cent had raised cholesterol levels.

There is also some evidence that a poor diet that is high in saturated fats and sugar and low in omega 3 fatty acids may contribute to a poorer prognosis and affect a person's recovery from schizophrenia (Peet, 2004). As such, it is vital for all nurses to be able to provide advice, support and guidance to people with mental health problems in terms of promoting healthy eating. Nurses need to ensure that their knowledge base is updated and that they have a working knowledge of the latest evidence relating to healthy eating. Wherever possible, they should seek to advise and guide people to consume a diet that will promote their physical health and overall well-being.

Exercise

The risks associated with an unhealthy diet are multiplied if a person does not engage in regular exercise. Inactivity increases the risk of obesity and type 2 diabetes. There is much evidence that people with mental health problems tend to be overweight when compared with the general population, and this is particularly pronounced among women (Kendrick, 1996), partly because they take less exercise. Brown et al. (1999) found in their study that a third of the people with mental health problems stated that they took no exercise at all. The symptoms of mental health problems (such as lethargy and poor motivation) and the side effects of some medication, such as sedation and weight gain (see below), can contribute to a poorer uptake of exercise as individuals may feel less able to become physically active.

Activity 4.5   *Critical thinking*

What do you feel might be the benefits of exercise for people with mental health problems?

An outline answer is given at the end of this chapter.

There is, however, much evidence that exercise can not only lead to improved physical health but also improve the symptoms of many mental health problems. Faulkner and Sparkes (1999), for example, found that a ten-week exercise programme for people diagnosed with schizophrenia led to improvements in the social, physical and psychological health of the participants. The National Institute for Health and Clinical Excellence (NICE) advise that physical activity programmes can be helpful to people experiencing mild to moderate depressive symptoms (NICE, 2007). Indeed, there are many physical gains in participating in exercise, such as improving body strength, sleep patterns, posture and flexibility. There are also psychosocial benefits, such as the tendency of physical activity to improve self-esteem and social contacts (Daley, 2002).

Medication

Psychiatric medication is widely used to treat a variety of mental health problems. While many people undoubtedly do benefit from the use of such medication, there is evidence that drugs used in mental health care can be associated with an increased risk to an individual's physical health, particularly when such drugs have been used over a long period of time. In particular, anti-psychotic medication, mood stabilisers and anti-depressants have been associated with weight gain (Robson and Gray, 2005, 2007) and diabetes (Citrome and Yeomans, 2005). Anti-psychotic medication can also affect the digestive system, liver, kidneys and circulatory system (Vanina et al., 2002). Some of the newer anti-psychotic medication (such as clozapine and olanzapine) has also been linked to the development of diabetes (Citrome and Yeomans, 2005) and hyper-lipidaemia (raised fat levels in the blood), which increase the risk of cardiovascular and cerebro-vascular disease (Koro et al., 2002). As mentioned above, it appears that some anti-psychotic medication can increase the hormone prolactin in the blood, disrupting menstruation and influencing fertility rates among young women. Furthermore, anti-psychotic medications have been linked to an increased risk of osteoporosis in this group (Halbreich and Palter, 1996).

Activity 4.6   *Communication*

Many drugs used in health care have side effects and it is important that you are able to help patients understand the risks and benefits of any medication regimen. How would you help a person to understand such risks and benefits? That is, how would you as a nurse ensure that the person is able to give properly informed consent to treatment with medicines?

An outline answer is given at the end of this chapter.

While it is important for nurses to understand the risks associated with medication that might undermine the physical health of people with mental health problems, this must be balanced against the benefits of their use for the individual in terms of their overall mental health and psychological well-being. Let us look at this in more depth by revisiting John's case discussed earlier in this chapter. There are clear benefits and risks associated with both taking and not taking medication. For example, medication that has sedating properties may affect John's breathing and may lead to him feeling unable or unwilling to undertake physical activity. His mood is low and he has not been attending to personal hygiene, increasing the risk of infections and dermatological problems. It is likely that John would be prescribed anti-depressant medication, which may lead to a number of side effects, such as retention of urine, constipation, headache, nausea and stomach upsets. For someone such as John who has a poor appetite, these side effects are unlikely to encourage him to eat. However, there is a real concern that John might be at risk of harming himself due to his low mood. Anti-depressant medication may be one way of assisting John to raise his mood, increasing his ability to self-care, exercise and make social contacts, and as his mood lifts, this may reduce the risk of self-harm.

Mental health problems

Stress, depression and social isolation can have a detrimental effect on the person's physical well-being. There is evidence, for example, that severe and chronic stress can have a detrimental impact on an individual's immunity, which increases their vulnerability to illness and disease (Tosevski and Milovancevic, 2006). In particular, stress is associated with the release into the body of proteins that have been linked to an increased risk of heart attacks, osteoporosis, arthritis, type 2 diabetes and some cancers (Ershler and Keller, 2000).

People with mental health problems also have an increased risk of misusing drugs and alcohol. The misuse of such substances carries a host of risks to an individual's physical health (including Hepatitis C and HIV/AIDS) and other associated risks such as violent behaviour and suicide, but they can also lead to a slower recovery from mental health problems (Vose, 2000).

As mentioned above, people diagnosed with schizophrenia demonstrate an increased risk of developing type 2 diabetes, and this risk is increased by lifestyle factors such as smoking, poor diet and a lack of exercise, along with the use of some forms of medication. However, for reasons that are not clear, there is an increased risk of diabetes among people diagnosed with schizophrenia who are not prescribed anti-psychotic medication (Ryan et al., 2003). There is a suggestion that factors that increase the risk of schizophrenia may also increase the risk of developing diabetes, and that this might be genetic (Mukherjee et al., 1989) as there is an increased rate of diabetes in the relatives of patients diagnosed with schizophrenia. However, it must be pointed out that even if there is a genetic predisposition for developing diabetes among people diagnosed with schizophrenia, this risk is likely to be exacerbated by the adoption of an unhealthy lifestyle (DRC, 2006).

Social and economic factors

Social support protects against the potential negative effects of both physical and mental health problems. However, it is vital to realise that the overall living conditions and the quality of social life that an individual experiences can also have a significant impact on health and well-being. People with mental health problems are more likely to live in areas with a general background of social deprivation, poor quality housing and high levels of crime, unemployment and drug misuse. They are also more at risk of being, or becoming, homeless when compared to the general population (Repper, 2000) and are more likely to experience social exclusion and poverty, factors that have been linked to poor health (Mentality/NIMHE, 2004). Within families, poor social support and high conflict between family members can have a detrimental impact on an individual's physical and mental health (Gilbert, 2006). You need to be aware of how such factors might apply to your individual patients and service users, and take steps wherever possible to assist them to improve their social well-being and living conditions and to ensure they are supported to return to work or to secure appropriate welfare benefits.

A holistic approach to health care

Let us look again at John's case. By looking more holistically we can determine that in addition to his physical health issues, John is experiencing significant issues in his psychological, social, emotional and spiritual dimensions of self. His diet is poor and he may not be able to intake sufficient quality nutrients. His energy levels suggest that he is not benefiting from regular exercise. He has reduced his social contacts, and his financial situation may impact on both his physical and mental well-being. The loss of his job has added significant stressors to his life – particularly financial. His job prospects seem to be poor, and he feels unable to provide for his family. This may have implications for how John sees his role within the family and may have an impact on his masculine identity. It appears that John is experiencing some symptoms of depression. Crucially, there may be a downward spiral here, where his low mood and depression may have a detrimental impact on the management of his asthma, which in turn may further lower his mood, which may have a detrimental impact on the management of his asthma and so on.

As such, our holistic understanding of John's mental and physical health issues, while adding a dimension of complexity, ultimately can reveal more useful insights into John's current situation. As a result, we as nurses are able to respond by targeting our helping responses to John's individual holistic needs. In helping John we need to consider the range of holistic measures that are available. As mentioned above, this includes medication – and here we need to support John to understand both the risks and benefits associated with psychiatric medication. Advice and support with regard to healthy eating and exercise may also be helpful to John, as would support to find meaningful work. We will discuss in more depth the nurse's role in helping people with mental health problems in Chapter 8.

Chapter summary

In this chapter we have looked at how physical and mental health might be linked. We have discussed how mental ill health may affect the prognosis of physical illness and disease and vice versa. We have also explored the factors that appear to increase the risk of physical illness and disease among a mental health service user group. We have discussed the importance for the nurse to recognise when apparent symptoms of mental ill health might be an indication of an underlying physical illness and to be mindful of the greater risk that this might pose for the ill person. We have also explored the holistic role of the nurse in ensuring that all patients are offered nursing care that improves their prognosis and recovery, and their overall health and well-being.

Activities: brief outline answers

Activity 4.1: Critical thinking (page 54)

Of course, there are wide individual variations in the response to any health issue but here you might have felt that physical illness affects us as follows.

- Physical – e.g. pain, lethargy, aches, fever.
- Social – withdrawal from friends and family, seeking reassurance from friends and family, joining support groups.
- Emotional – anxiety, worry, stress, sadness, grief, fear.
- Psychological – thoughts about self and ability to cope, loss of control, thoughts that one is a burden.
- Spiritual – reflections on the future, reflecting on the meaning of the disease.

Activity 4.2: Evidence-based practice (page 56)

There are many possible reasons here. One might be because the person is exposed to a great number of risk factors (such as lifestyle factors highlighted later in the chapter). There is also a possibility that medication that is used to treat mental health problems might lead to the development of physical health problems or exacerbate an existing condition. Sometimes a person may not engage with health care services or may not report symptoms so that they can be treated at an early stage. However, there is also some evidence that the physical health care needs of people with mental health problems may not be taken seriously, leading to poorer access to medical care and surgical treatment.

Activity 4.3: Critical thinking (page 58)

- Nicotine might act to alleviate some of the symptoms of mental health problems and the side effects of medication.
- Nicotine can be relaxing when one is stressed or energising when one is feeling tired and lethargic.
- Physiological addiction.
- Social reasons.
- Pleasure.
- Smoking may be considered to be a part of the mental health culture and useful to the development of a therapeutic relationship – and therefore not challenged by nurses.
- A lack of smoking cessation advice offered by nurses and other health care professionals.

Activity 4.4: Critical thinking (page 59)

It is recommended that a person consumes a weekly minimum of five portions of fruit or vegetables each day and one portion of oily fish (DH, 2004c). Diets should be low in salt, high in vitamins and nutrients, fibre and omega 3 fatty acids. However, there is likely to be considerable variation here in terms of personal preferences and religious observances, and also in terms of an individual's tolerances for particular types of food based on allergies and health conditions.

Activity 4.5: Critical thinking (page 59)

The obvious benefit is that exercise can lead to improved physical health, body strength, sleep patterns, posture and flexibility. There are also psychosocial benefits, such as the tendency of physical activity to improve self-esteem and social contacts. However, exercise can also improve the symptoms of many mental health problems; it has been shown to be helpful to people experiencing mild to moderate depressive symptoms and has led to improvements in the social, physical and psychological health in people diagnosed with schizophrenia.

Activity 4.6: Communication (page 60)

This question is concerned with the promotion of informed consent. At first glance, it appears that medication used in mental health care is extremely dangerous. However, this is not the case, as all drugs prescribed in psychiatry are safe for human use and have been subjected to rigorous testing before a licence is issued. However, nurses must be mindful that intolerable side effects are often associated with poor adherence. Here, it is vital that the nurse shares with the patient their knowledge of side effects in order to assist their patients to be aware and watchful of them, and they must encourage their patients to report any unwanted effects at the first opportunity. The patient should be reminded that there are risks and benefits associated with any medication. If the nurse feels that such discussions exceed their own knowledge and understanding, then they should ensure that the prescriber is contacted for further information and advice.

Further reading

Blows, W (2011) *The biological basis of mental health nursing.* London: Routledge.

This is an excellent book that explores the biological basis of mental health problems.

Margereson, C and Trenoweth, S (2010) *Developing holistic care for long-term conditions.* London: Routledge.

This book illustrates how a holistic approach can be taken across a wide range of long-term conditions, including mental health problems.

Nash, M (2010) *Physical health and well-being in mental health nursing.* Oxford: Oxford University Press.

This is a comprehensive book that highlights the skills needed to provide physical health care to people experiencing mental health problems.

Chapter 5
Legal and ethical issues in mental health nursing

Terry Docherty

NMC Standards for Pre-registration Nursing Education

This chapter will address the following competencies:

Domain 1: Professional values

1.1. **Mental health nurses** must understand and apply current legislation to all service users, paying special attention to the protection of vulnerable people, including those with complex needs arising from ageing, cognitive impairment, long-term conditions and those approaching the end of life.

2.1. **Mental health nurses** must practise in a way that addresses the potential power imbalances between professionals and people experiencing mental health problems, including situations when compulsory measures are used, by helping people exercise their rights, upholding safeguards and ensuring minimal restrictions on their lives. They must have an in depth understanding of mental health legislation and how it relates to care and treatment of people with mental health problems.

NMC Essential Skills Clusters

This chapter will address the following ESCs:

Cluster: Care, compassion and communication

1. As partners in the care process, people can trust a newly registered graduate nurse to provide collaborative care based on the highest standards, knowledge and competence.

By the first progression point:

1. Articulates the underpinning values of *The code: standards of conduct, performance and ethics for nurses and midwives* (the Code) (NMC, 2008a).

4. Shows respect for others.

2. People can trust the newly registered graduate nurse to engage in person centred care empowering people to make choices about how their needs are met when they are unable to meet them for themselves.

continued overleaf . . .

continued . . . ●●●

By entry to the register:
9. Ensures access to independent advocacy.
10. Recognises situations and acts appropriately when a person's choice may compromise their safety or the safety of others.

4. People can trust a newly qualified graduate nurse to engage with them and their family or carers within their cultural environments in an acceptant and anti-discriminatory manner free from harassment and exploitation.

By the first progression point:
2. Respects people's rights.
3. Adopts a principled approach to care underpinned by the Code (NMC, 2008a).

7. People can trust the newly registered graduate nurse to protect and keep as confidential all information relating to them.

By the first progression point:
1. Applies the principles of confidentiality.
2. Protects and treats information as confidential except where sharing information is required for the purposes of safeguarding and public protection.
3. Applies the principles of data protection.

8. People can trust the newly registered graduate nurse to gain their consent based on sound understanding and informed choice prior to any intervention and that their rights in decision making and consent will be respected and upheld.

By the first progression point:
1. Seeks consent prior to sharing confidential information outside of the professional care team, subject to agreed safeguarding and protection procedures.

By the second progression point:
2. Applies principles of consent in relation to restrictions relating to specific client groups and seeks consent for care.
3. Ensures that the meaning of consent to treatment and care is understood by the people or service users.

Organisational aspects of care
11. People can trust the newly registered graduate nurse to safeguard children and adults from vulnerable situations and support and protect them from harm.

By the first progression point:
1. Acts within legal frameworks and local policies in relation to safeguarding adults and children who are in vulnerable situations.
2. Shares information with colleagues and seeks advice from appropriate sources where there is a concern or uncertainty.

By the second progression point:
4. Documents concerns and information about people who are in vulnerable situations.

Chapter aims

By the end of this chapter, you should be able to:

* outline the subject of ethics in nursing;
* describe the legal system in the UK;
* outline the role and function of the NMC;
* recognise the main legislation that affects people with mental health problems;
* discuss ways of safeguarding service users.

Introduction

All nurses are bound by the laws of the land and professionally by *The code: standards of conduct, performance and ethics for nurses and midwives* (NMC, 2008a) – the Code. Nurses working with people who have mental health problems are often faced with situations for which knowledge of both the law and ethics is essential. This chapter will explore the ethical and legal aspects of caring for people with mental health problems. We will look at the subject of ethics in general and nursing ethics in particular, and outline the main ethical perspectives. The chapter will go on to discuss what law is, how laws are made, and how they apply to nurses. We will also look at the structure, purpose and functions of the NMC. Finally, we will discuss the main areas of legislation that relate to caring for the mentally ill and the measures available for safeguarding.

What is ethics?

There are many definitions of ethics; here are some of them.

Ethics is concerned with the study and practice of what is good and right for human beings.
(Thompson et al., 2000)

Ethics is the study of morals in human conduct, the rules of conduct recognised as appropriate to a particular profession or area of life.
(*Oxford English Reference Dictionary*, 1996)

Ethics is a branch philosophy that deals with the distinction between right and wrong, with moral consequences of human actions.
(*Stedman's Medical Dictionary*, 2000)

Ethics is the science or study of moral values or principles, including ideals of autonomy, beneficence and justice.
(*Mosby's Medical Nursing and Allied Health Dictionary*, 2000)

As we can see from the definitions above, ethics is referred to as the study of morals, but what are morals? The distinction between the two is not clear: 'morals' comes from the Latin *moralis* meaning custom, manner or law, and 'ethics' comes from the Greek *ethikos* meaning custom or usage. In practice the words ethics and morals are used interchangeably. According to Rumbold (1999) ethics is a branch of philosophy, and while philosophy is concerned with macro issues such as the meaning of life, ethics is concerned more with human actions and the value of these actions. So we can think of ethics as rules for behaviour, which for some of us stem from our religious beliefs; others would say it is doing what the law requires, or the standards of behaviour that our society accepts. Ethics does not provide neat answers to all situations, but it does give us a means to explain and justify our actions and helps us clarify the moral values that determine our actions. As in ordinary life, nursing is full of situations where moral choices have to be made; such situations involve not only what you do but also what you do not do. Those involved in providing health care are faced with a range of challenges, including caring for people whose lifestyle and values are different from their own and caring for people in compulsory detention. New treatments and technologies offer hope and new ways of treating individuals, but there is the problem of deciding who should have access to these new and often expensive forms of treatment.

Activity 5.1 *Reflection*

Can you identify any forms of treatment where an ethical dilemma would occur? Consider your own values. What are your set of values and the moral rules that you hold dear? How do you think you came to have these values, in particular, rather than any other values? Did you always have these values?

As this is an individual reflection, there is no outline answer at the end of the chapter.

Ethics in nursing

What values did you list in Activity 5.1? Perhaps you value truthfulness or believe that we should always help those who are in need. Others may value success and admit that cunning and trickery are essential in gaining success in life. Still others believe that rules and laws do not matter so long as you are not caught breaking them. Share the findings of this exercise with your friends or colleagues and you will probably find that not everyone has the same values as you. The fact that we hold different values in some ways explains the difficulties we have in reaching agreements in day-to-day life. When you are caring for patients you will be confronted with difficult situations that may often challenge your own values and standards. If you have an understanding of ethics, it can help you to explain and justify your decision making when faced with the dilemmas of difficult situations, and also help you identify your own values. Further, viewing a situation from an ethical perspective helps the process of reflection, which may prompt us to rethink or pause before taking action that may unwittingly be callous or insensitive. Let us look at the kind of situations you will encounter where ethical judgements need to be made.

Ethical principles applied to nursing

When you are a registered nurse, the NMC standards require you to conduct yourself and to deliver care within an **ethical framework**. In order to use a framework you need to understand ethical principles. Most writers on ethics would agree that there are four key ethical principles.

1. Respect for autonomy (the individual's right to make their own decisions).
2. Non-maleficence (do no harm).
3. Beneficence (doing good).
4. Justice (should prescribe actions that are fair to those involved).
   (Beauchamp and Childress, 2001)

These four principles can be seen at work in nursing, and we will now look at each of them in turn to see how these principles apply in working with people who have mental health problems.

Autonomy

The concept of autonomy stems from the work of the German philosopher Immanuel Kant (1724–1804), who argued that the concept of 'the person' is central for the existence of ethics and that the individual is the bearer of rights. The word 'autonomy' comes from the Greek *autos* = self and *nomos* = law, and while we should never be a law unto ourselves, we do live in a society with a fair degree of personal freedom and few of the external constraints found in many other societies. For example, we have freedom of movement, of expression and to live generally in a manner that suits us in matters such as diet. These freedoms are individual rights, and over the years these rights have been added to; a recent example is the right of same-sex couples to enter into civil partnerships with the same legal rights as marriage. Rights can also be taken away, for example, the right to smoke in public places. As a nurse you must respect the autonomy of each individual patient, and this means that you will:

* seek consent for many aspects of care, especially those that involve physical touch;
* inform the patient about their treatment and what being cared for may entail;
* be an advocate for the patient, supporting their views, especially when they are unable to express their feelings.

Preserving the autonomy of a patient with mental illness is one of the most challenging issues for those caring for the mentally ill. The mentally ill are often detained against their will, and, further, they may receive treatment they do not agree with, such as rapid tranquillisation or seclusion. Those caring for the mentally ill have a duty to respond to difficult situations where action has to be taken to avoid danger to the patient. For example, a patient's judgement may be influenced by **delusional** ideas – reinforced by auditory hallucinations – that other individuals are trying to harm them, so much so they feel they have to threaten or physically assault others. Conversely, many of those with mental health problems require protection from society, for example, individuals with **dementia** or those whose behaviour may arouse hostility or derision in others. This need for protection could also apply to those with physical conditions such as thyroid problems or the development of space-occupying lesions in the brain, or to those in acute confessional states brought on by a chest infection. Another example would be an individual who, due to his delusional ideas, feels he deserves to die and so refuses to eat or drink, resulting in life-threatening dehydration. This is a situation that would call for us to treat the individual against their wishes. So while we are breaching an individual's right of autonomy we are arguably acting ethically in preventing harm to the individual. Here the principle of beneficence is the ethical underpinning of our decision making, and we can see that using ethics enables us to explain and justify our actions.

Non-maleficence

Non-maleficence is the principle of doing no harm. There are circumstances in caring for those with a mental illness where not taking action may be the most ethically appropriate position to adopt. For example, many would argue that those caring for the mentally ill should exercise caution in detaining service users in hospital against their will and in the giving of a psychiatric diagnosis. Some of you will be saying that giving treatment to those who suffer from mental health problems is what mental health services are about. However, while detaining someone in a mental health hospital and giving them a diagnosis may appear outwardly to be for that individual's good, there may be long-term adverse consequences, for example, in areas such as gaining employment, emigration or obtaining insurance or a loan. Once a diagnosis is given or the individual is detained in hospital under the Mental Health Act this becomes a matter of record and exposes the individual to risk of stigma and isolation (Dawson and Szmukler, 2006). Care needs to be taken in making these decisions, and where possible in the case of detaining an individual, all efforts should made to avoid its use. A brief look at the history of caring for the mentally ill will provide many examples of care and treatment that did little to help those with mental health problems.

Beneficence

Beneficence means doing good, and while most people would agree that doing good is a worthwhile aim, there are occasions where in our efforts to do good we are actually doing the opposite. A nurse making decisions on behalf of the patient, believing it is in their best interests, is adopting a 'paternalistic' approach, and in doing so may lessen the individual's ability to make decisions for themselves, making them ill-equipped to function independently. However, there are many situations where the individual has lost the capacity to make rational decisions; for example, they may have **paranoid** delusions in which they feel they are at risk from others. This inability to make clear decisions and to accurately assess their environment can result in actions that could cause harm to themselves and others. Here, it may be in the best interests of the individual to restrict their movement and detain them in a mental health setting. While this could be seen as infringing the autonomy of the individual, the action can be ethically justified as being for their greater good. This would be an example of 'paternalistic beneficence' – the decision making is for the good of the individual.

Justice

Justice refers to the ethical duty to treat people fairly and not to discriminate against them. This may seem very straightforward and many would argue that they would do this as a matter of course. However, in the course of caring for individuals with a mental illness – or, indeed, a physical illness – you will meet people whose moral values and way of life will challenge your own. It may be easier and more enjoyable to care for people you like and find interesting, but you will be expected to provide a similar quality of care to those whose views and lifestyles are very different from your own. Let us look at the kind of situation you will encounter where ethical judgements need to be made.

Activity 5.2 — Decision making

1. A patient tells you that they have not been taking their medication all the time, but asks you not to tell the rest of the clinical staff.
2. Later that day, you are offered a very expensive gift from the family of a patient you are looking after.
3. The next morning, a female patient confides in you that she is a lesbian.

Reflect on these situations and consider what action you should take in each case.

There is no outline answer at the end of the chapter, but some discussion on how ethical principles and the NMC Code (NMC, 2008a) may help to shape and support your decision making is set out below.

In the first situation in Activity 5.2 the patient clearly feels the need to tell someone that they are not taking their medication, and you should explore the reason for their refusal to take medication. What ethical principle will underpin your actions? This patient is informal in that they are not legally detained in hospital and can refuse treatment should they wish. So, by not sharing this with the rest of the team, you may be respecting the autonomy of the patient. However, this course of action may not be in the interests of the patient. Sharing the information could be seen as beneficence – you are doing good by ensuring the patient continues with their treatment. On the other hand, you may have built up a trusting relationship, and sharing the information might do harm by confirming in the patient's mind that no one can be trusted.

It would seem best to inform the patient that you are professionally bound to act in the best interests of the patient, which may require you to share the information. The patient may welcome a suggestion that together you speak to the medical team about this matter.

With regard to the second situation in the activity, the Code clearly states: *You must refuse any gifts, favours or hospitality that might be interpreted as an attempt to gain preferential treatment* (NMC, 2008a). However, it goes on to say: *Nurses and midwives can receive gifts or favours from people they care for but must be confident that the giving of these gifts could not be interpreted as being in return for preferential treatment.* The key word is 'preferential' – the nurse may find themselves in a situation where they are expected to give better care to this patient. If the nurse does give care that is not of the same standard as that given to others, this is clearly unethical under the principle of equity. Some Trusts have rules about what nurses can receive, and usually limit gifts to a relatively small sum of money – say, £10. Another point to consider is that the gift may not be about you and what you, in particular, have done, but rather about the position you hold.

In the third situation a patient has shared very sensitive information with you, which would indicate a level of trust. You will need to ask why she felt the need to share the information and the team? If she wishes only you to know, then it would be in keeping with the principle of autonomy that you do not share this information. However, it could be that she is having difficulties in coming to terms with her sexuality and that this has a bearing on her current mental health problems. If so, to do good (beneficence), you should be urging the patient to share the information with others.

The judicial system in England and Wales

In this section we will be looking at what law is and how laws are made in this country. Law covers virtually all aspects of living and dying; it provides standards of behaviour without which our society could not successfully function. Moreover, as our society becomes more complex, so do its laws. 'Law' can be described as 'rules' or 'a collection of rules', a rule being defined as an authoritative regulation or direction concerning method (*Collins dictionary*, 2001, p1313). For example, it is a criminal offence for someone to portray themselves as a registered nurse when they are not.

How UK law is made

Two main forces shape the development of law: common law (also known as case law or judge-made law), which results from the decisions made on legal cases, and statutory provision, such as Acts of Parliament.

Common law

Common law is malleable; it evolves to meet the changing needs of society and its improved level of understanding. An example of the impact of common law arose from the case of *Gillick v West Norfolk and Wisbech Area Health Authority* [1985] 3 All ER 402 (HL). In this case Victoria Gillick objected to the practice of prescribing contraception to girls under the age of 16 without their parents' permission. The case went to the House of Lords, which found in favour of the health authority, and from this ruling it was decided that:

> *whether or not a child is capable of giving the necessary consent will depend on the child's maturity and understanding and the nature of the consent required. The child must be capable of making a reasonable assessment of the advantages and disadvantages of the treatment proposed, so the consent, if given, can be properly and fairly described as true consent.*
> (Lord Scarman, Lord Fraser and Lord Bridge in the case cited above)

This case established Gillick competence, which became a legally accepted method of deciding whether an under-16 year old could give their consent. Gillick competence has now been replaced by the Fraser guidelines. For further information on Gillick competence and the Fraser guidelines, please consult **www.nspcc.org.uk/inform/research/questions/gillick_wda61289.html**.

Statutory law

The idea for a new law can come from a number of sources, including government-generated policy, pressure groups, the influence of experts within their field and an EU directive. A new law must go through a number of stages. First, the government publishes a Green Paper to introduce the subject to the public and interested parties for consultation and to stimulate wider discussion, with no commitment for action. The government then issues a White Paper, which sets out the proposed legislative changes, giving the public a clear idea of the specific proposals. While a White Paper is mainly about informing the public about the direction of government policy and to stimulate discussion, it is normally debated in parliament as a bill. Once the legislative changes have been passed by both houses of parliament, the bill becomes law.

Criminal law and civil law

The law in England and Wales is divided into criminal law and civil law. There are a number of differences (see Table 5.1), but generally criminal law involves the rules laid down by the state for citizens, while civil law governs the relationships and transactions between citizens.

As you can see in Table 5.1, the burden of proof is less in civil cases and legal advice may recommend taking civil action rather than criminal action as there is a greater likelihood of a successful outcome.

Criminal	**Civil**
The offence is against the state	The offence is against the individual
Proof of guilt has to be beyond reasonable doubt	Liability is on the balance of probabilities
Outcome: fines, prison, absolute discharge	Outcome: compensation, in the form of an apology or financial remuneration

Table 5.1: Criminal law and civil law

> ### Activity 5.4 _Critical thinking_
>
> Ann is a 27-year-old nurse who is the nurse in charge on night duty with two other members of staff. A female patient returns to the ward smelling of alcohol; she also has an injury to her skull and there is evidence of slight bleeding. The patient is examined by the doctor on duty for that evening, who says that the patient is to be closely observed and kept on regular neurological observations. Ann delegates the care to the two junior nurses. Later, the patient is found to be in a coma and dies shortly afterwards. The subsequent investigation finds that the quality of nursing care was substandard, in that the level of observation was poor and neurological observations had not been carried out.
>
> What are the legal and professional implications of this situation?
>
> *An outline answer is given at the end of the chapter.*

The role of the NMC and nursing as a profession

> ### Activity 5.5 _Reflection_
>
> Before reading further, consider what you think is the main function and purpose of the NMC and make notes for yourself. At the end of this section compare your original thoughts in the light of what you have learned.
>
> *An outline answer is given at the end of the chapter.*

The development of the Nursing and Midwifery Council (NMC)

The first professional body for nurses was the General Nursing Council (GNC), set up after the passing of the Nurses Registration Act of 1919. The GNC continued until 1983 when it became the United Kingdom Central Council for Nursing, Midwifery and Health Visiting (UKCC). The UKCC brought together the various councils that represented nursing throughout the UK, so for the first time there was a national register of nurses in the UK. The UKCC was also required to monitor the quality of educational training for nurses: four National Boards were set up, one for each part of the UK. The UKCC was replaced by the Nursing and Midwifery Council (NMC) in 2002 with the passing of the Nursing and Midwifery Order (2001), which gave the NMC statutory powers to monitor standards of education, training, conduct and performance. The establishment of the NMC brought together for the first time the functions of registering nurses, the handling of professional misconduct and the monitoring of nursing and midwifery educational courses. The NMC is the professional body that all nurses must be registered with if they wish to practise as a nurse in the UK.

Before we go on to look at the role and function of the NMC, let us consider what it is to be a professional. In the past, what was considered a profession was limited to medicine, law and Church ministry. Nowadays, the term is used more widely of a broader range of occupations, but ones that have aspects in common.

Activity 5.6   *Reflection*

Make a list of reasons why you think nursing is a profession.

An outline answer is given at the end of the chapter.

As a nurse you may be surprised at the expectations people have of you. For some, being a nurse is more than just a job, and different from, say, working in an office. They see nursing as a vocation, a 'calling', maybe with an element of self-sacrifice. While others see this as an old-fashioned view, the reality is that nursing is a profession, and one in which nurses are being trained to take on greater responsibility in the treatment and care of patients. Moreover, nurses are taking on roles that were once reserved for doctors; for example, a growing number of nurses are prescribing medicine.

The question of what defines a profession is an area of constant debate that has attracted a number of writers. Good (1960) states that a profession has two core characteristics: a prolonged specific training with a body of abstract knowledge, and a service orientation or a collectively involving internal regulation and agreement about what it is doing. Eliot Friedson identified four key characteristics of a profession.

1. Adherence to a code of ethics.
2. Professional autonomy: the power of the profession to define and control its own work.
3. Specialised knowledge, added to by research.
4. A monopoly, where the professionals (and they only) do this type of work.
    1970, cited in Blane, 1991

Reeves and Orford (2002) define a profession as *an occupation that possesses a specific body of knowledge that is in the main unique from that of other professions*. Moreover, a profession requires a lengthy period of education and development that includes the support and assessment by members of that profession. So, for an activity to be called a profession there has to be a body of special knowledge unique to this group, a period of training, evidence of ethical practice and that they, and only they, carry out this activity or work.

A professional is defined as an individual who is extremely competent in a job or basically very good at what they do. Hoyle and John's (1995) definition of the professional can be summarised as one who applies expert or specialist knowledge, is capable of autonomous thought and judgement, and has a responsibility to clients and the wider society through voluntary commitment to a set of principles. Professionalisation refers to the process of development that a trade or activity goes through in order to become a recognised profession (Hunt and Wainwright, 1994, p6).

We will now go on the look at some definitions of nursing to see how they compare with our understanding of a profession. This is how the International Council of Nurses (2010) defined nursing:

> *Nursing encompasses autonomous and collaborative care of individuals of all ages, families, groups and communities, sick or well and in all settings. Nursing includes the promotion of health, prevention of illness, and the care of ill, disabled and dying people. Advocacy, promotion of a safe environment, research, participation in shaping health policy and in patient and health systems management, and education are also key nursing roles.*

A more detailed view of nursing comes from the Royal College of Nursing in their report *Defining Nursing* (RCN, 2003b) which distinguished professional nursing as:

- the clinical judgement inherent in the processes of assessment, diagnosis, prescription and evaluation;
- the knowledge that is the basis of the assessment of need and the determination of action to meet the need;
- the personal accountability for all decisions and actions, including the decision to delegate to others the structured relationship between the nurse and the patient, which incorporates professional regulation and a code of ethics within a statutory framework.

A number of writers have questioned the professional status of nursing. Etzioni (1969) identified occupations such as nursing, teaching and social work as semi-professions, pointing out that their training is shorter, with a less specialised body of knowledge and limited autonomy. Support for this view comes from Sleicher (1981) and Feldman (1981) who both maintained that nursing lacks a sufficient body of knowledge. Liaschoenko and Peter (2004) question the level of autonomous activity of nurses and make the point that nurses are subordinate to the agendas set by other professions. However, the title 'Registered Nurse' is protected by law, and the requirements to be a registered nurse are set out in statute law (Nurses, Midwives and Health Visitors Act 1997). Further, nurses are expanding their practice with developments in areas such as applying psycho-social interventions and nurse prescribing. Moreover, nurses have to undergo a lengthy period of training, which will soon be available at degree level only. The position of nursing as a profession is strengthened by the requirement of the NMC Code (2008a) that places a clear responsibility for registered nurses *to facilitate students and others to develop* (Number 23); and *you must be willing to share your skills and experience* (Number 25). The Code requires nurses to make the care of people their first concern: *the nurse recognises the need for accountability . . . placing the needs of a patient/client before that of their profession*. It is fair to say that there is an ongoing debate regarding the professional status of nursing.

The role of the NMC

The role of the NMC is to safeguard the health and well-being of the public.

Activity 5.7   *Reflection*

The NMC has a range of measures in place to safeguard the public. How do they go about this? Use the following link: **www.nmc-uk.org/About-us/Our-role/**

An outline answer is given at the end of the chapter.

In putting ourselves in the care of others, we trust that the skills and knowledge of the clinicians are appropriate for the procedure we are about to undergo and that we will be well looked after. Unfortunately, there are occasions where care is not at an acceptable level or a patient is badly treated due to their vulnerability. To protect the public from poor or substandard care the NMC maintains a register of nurses who have undergone a recognised period of education and development at a level set by the NMC; only these registered nurses are allowed to use the title Registered Nurse. The NMC Code (2008a) also requires nurses to consider how they will conduct themselves in both their personal and professional lives. It is this Code with which you will need to be familiar throughout your nursing career.

Activity 5.8   *Reflection*

Go to **www.nmc-uk.org**, then open 'Publications' and then 'Standards' and select *The code: Standards of conduct, performance and ethics for nurses and midwives.* Listen to the Code being read out to you. Consider the impact the Code will have upon you, both in your professional and personal life.

As this activity is based on your own reflection, there is no outline answer.

As discussed above, the NMC Code (2008a) requires a nurse to work within an ethical framework; nurses are also bound by the laws of the land and must conduct themselves accordingly. The Nursing and Midwifery Order (2001) sets out in statute that to practise as a nurse the individual must meet current standards as laid down by the NMC; further, the nurse must be of 'good character'. While only 0.2 per cent of the nursing population of 663,656 (in March 2009) is referred to the NMC for misconduct, the overall trend is upwards. Referrals from the public doubled to 16.8 per cent in the year 2008–09 compared to 8.8 per cent in 2007–08. The latest figures from the NMC show that the number of referrals has increased from 1,478 in 2007–08 to 2,988 for the period 2009–10 (NMC, 2009, Table 13). All nurses are bound by the Code *to adhere to the laws of the country in which you are practising* (NMC, 2008a, Number 49). Further, the Code (Number 50) requires all nurses to inform the NMC if they have been cautioned, charged or found guilty of an offence. You are required by Number 51 of the Code to inform your employers if your fitness to practise has been questioned. If a nurse is convicted of any criminal offence, whether it relates to nursing or not, the police are required to inform the NMC; they are also required to tell the NMC if a nurse has received a caution. Out of 2,988 referrals to the NMC during 2009–10, 576 came from the police (NMC, 2009, Table 13). The NMC has Fitness for Practice committees with the power to sanction a nurse, such as giving a caution.

Nurses and midwives can be referred to the NMC if there are concerns about their fitness to practise or for any of the following reasons: misconduct; lack of competence; a conviction or caution (including a finding of guilt by a court martial); physical or mental ill health; a finding by any other health or social care regulator or licensing body that a nurse or midwife's fitness to practise is impaired, or a barring under the arrangements provided by the Safeguarding Vulnerable Groups Act 2006, the Safeguarding Vulnerable Groups (Northern Ireland) Order 2007 or the Protection of Vulnerable Groups (Scotland) Act 2007 (NMC, 2010c).

Once an allegation is made it is prioritised according to the severity of the allegation, and an investigation committee will assess if there is a case to answer. If there is no case to answer, the matter will end there and the nurse will not have to answer the complaint made against them. If there is a case, then depending on the circumstances, a referral will go for a decision (adjudication) to the Conduct and Competence Committee or the Health Committee.

Following the NMC adjudication, the panel hearing the case can apply one of a number of sanctions as set out in Table 5.2. As the main purpose of the sanctions is to protect the public, a decision may also include identifying future training and development for the nurse in question.

Interim orders

In cases where there has been a serious assault or the nurse is considered a danger to the public if they remain in clinical practice, an interim order hearing is arranged as soon as possible, and the registrant can be suspended for up to 18 months while the investigation into the allegation continues. The following box gives examples of cases that have been referred to the NMC and their outcomes.

Case studies

A mental health nurse was reported to the NMC for breach of patient confidentiality. He divulged personal information about a patient that he received from a colleague; the breach resulted in considerable distress for the patient and his family. Following a hearing by the Conduct and Competence Committee, the allegations were proven and he was given a caution for two years.

A female nurse was found to be intoxicated while responsible for a large group of vulnerable mental health patients where there was a potential for a serious risk of harm. From the reports submitted to the panel it appeared that this was not an isolated occurrence, so an interim suspension order of 18 months was given while further medical reports were sought.

A female mental nurse was given an interim suspension of 18 months and later struck off the register as she was found to be repeatedly taking time off, which she claimed was due to sickness. During these periods of reported sickness she secured work as a nurse in other health care settings. She provided many references of good character, but the panel decision was influenced by a previous finding against this nurse when she received a caution for five years for giving false information about her manager during an investigation.

*If you wish to see further outcomes of cases of misconduct, go to the NMC website (**www.nmc-uk.org**), then follow to the link to 'Hearings' and then 'Outcomes'.*

Legal aspects of nursing

Consent

Caring for people with mental health problems will place you in situations that are at times puzzling and difficult to understand. For example, an individual may refuse treatment that you

Decision	Time	Rationale
Take no further action		
Caution the registrant and direct that the caution be noted against the registrant's entry in the register for a period of not less than one and not more than five years (a caution order)	1 to 5 years	There is evidence that behaviour would not have caused direct or indirect harm to a patient. There is early admission of facts alleged and/or an insight into failings; it is an isolated incident that was not deliberate. There is genuine expression of regret or an apology; the registrant was acting under duress. There is previous good history, no reoccurrence; corrective steps have been taken; there are positive references or testimonials.
Impose conditions with which the registrant must comply for a specified period of not more than three years (a conditions of practice order). For example: *The Registrant shall not have any financial dealings nor have access to or handle any patient or employee money or The Registrant shall not administer medication or hold the drug keys.*	3 years, but may be reviewed	Identifiable areas of the registrant's practice are in need of retraining and there is no evidence of general incompetence (lack of competence cases). There is the potential and a willingness to respond positively to conditions requiring retraining (misconduct and lack of competence cases). There is a willingness to comply with conditions requiring supervision of health (health cases). The conditions will protect patients and clients during the period they are in force.

Table 5.2: Sanctions available to the NMC

Decision	Time	Rationale
Suspend the individual's registration for a period of up to one year (a suspension order)	1 year but may be reviewed	There has been misconduct, but not misconduct that is fundamentally incompatible with continuing to be registered with the NMC. There is an apparently irremediable lack of competence but striking-off is not available. The registrant has serious ill health but striking-off is not available.
Strike the individual off the register (a striking-off order)		There has been a serious departure from the relevant standards as set out in *The code: Standards of conduct performance and ethics for nurses and midwives* or other NMC standards, and/or where there is continuing risk to patients, clients or others. The registrant's behaviour would undermine confidence in the NMC if they were not struck off. There has been a serious lack of competence where there is no evidence of improvement following two years of continuous suspension or conditions of practice.

Table 5.2: Continued

see as helping them or indeed saving their life. There are many possible reasons for such a refusal – a bad previous experience of health care or fear of the treatment itself, for instance. Whatever the reasons, if a patient is mentally competent we have to accept their right to refuse treatment. The main ethical reason for obtaining patient consent is to protect the patient's autonomy. As we discussed earlier, autonomy is the right to self-determination, where an individual can decide for themselves what they want to happen in their lives. While many nursing interventions would not be described as major procedures, they can still be 'morally significant' to the patient, and not getting the patient's informed consent could be a serious infringement of their autonomy. Examples of such procedures are helping with personal hygiene and giving injections; patients should have a say in when these are done, and have the procedures explained to them. Moreover, they should also feel free to ask for clarification on any of the procedures you are carrying out.

Later, we will look at what 'mentally competent' means, but for now we will examine informed consent, and the legal and ethical aspects of giving consent. The Code (NMC, 2008a) places a clear responsibility upon nurses to obtain informed consent to treatment. More recently this has been emphasised with publications such as *Safeguarding adults and the NHS* (2011). Gaining the consent of a patient to treatment is implicit throughout the Code, and sections 13 to 17 clearly direct nurses to channel their energy and efforts not only at gaining consent from the patient but also in assisting the patient to make decisions about their treatment that they understand and are in agreement with. The Code states:

13. *You must ensure that you gain consent before you begin any treatment or care.*
14. *You must respect and support people's rights to accept or decline treatment and care.*
15. *You must uphold people's rights to be fully involved in decisions about their care.*
16. *You must be aware of the legislation regarding mental capacity, ensuring that people who lack capacity remain at the centre of decision making and are fully safeguarded.*
17. *You must be able to demonstrate that you have acted in someone's best interests if you have provided care in an emergency.*

(NMC, 2008a)

In law, there are three recognised ways in which consent can be given (Dimond, 2008). First, there is written consent – the patient signs a statement that they consent to an examination or treatment. The Department of Health has produced forms for consent in its *Reference guide to consent for examination or treatment* (DH, 2009b), but Trusts remain free to develop their own documentation. Consent can also be given verbally; here the patient will agree to be examined. Such agreement can be implied, for example, by rolling up their sleeve to have an injection. Aveyard (2002) urges nurses to be cautious here, as gaining the patient's willingness, without giving information, could more accurately be called **compliance**. Failing to obtain consent could result in legal action being taken against you. For example, touching or examining a patient without their permission could be viewed as battery, or failing to fully inform a patient about their care and treatment could be seen as a breach of the nurse's duty of care. Let us now look at what we mean by informed consent.

Activity 5.9   *Communication*

Here are examples of things that nurses sometimes say that may put patients under duress to comply with treatment. Can you think of some more?

- If you don't take this medication, we will have to give you an injection.
- You have to make your mind up now as I am very busy.

Further examples are provided at the end of the chapter.

Beauchamp and Childress (2001) state that informed consent *occurs if and only if a patient or subject with substantial understanding and in substantial absence of control by others intentionally authorizes a professional to do something* (p143). We may seem to have obtained a patient's cooperation for treatment, but this may not include their agreement, and while they may be informed, their acceptance may not be entirely voluntary. For many, finding themselves in a mental health hospital can be a stressful and frightening experience, resulting in feeling intimidated by the strangeness of their new situation and unwilling to express their true feelings; their decision to accept treatment may be out of deference to clinical staff.

Considering the ethical and legal perspectives of informed consent, from a moral perspective informed consent is about giving the individual autonomy, helping them to make a decision by making sure they understand the consequences. From a legal perspective, the issue of informed consent is largely concerned with removing the likelihood of civil litigation.

According to Beauchamp and Childress (2001) informed consent consists of two elements: the giving of information, which requires the disclosure of information and the comprehension of that information; and voluntary consent – there is agreement to undergo a medical procedure or treatment. While the Code expects that you obtain informed consent and share with the patient information that they want or need to know, the amount and depth of information disclosed may vary according to the clinical setting. Indeed, the term 'informed consent' has been criticised as jargonistic and lacking clarity.

There are two main schools of thought about what information should be disclosed to patients. The professional practice standard is the one that exists in a particular clinical area; for example, patients may be informed about a number of the side effects of medication but not all. Further variations include how the information is given; it may be verbal in one setting and written in another. This approach is open to criticism as there is no national standard, and clinical staff may lack the skills to decide what is in the best interests of the patient. Indeed, having a professional standard undermines autonomous decision making. The other approach is the 'reasonable person' standard, which places greater emphasis on autonomous decision making than the rather paternalistic beneficence of the professional practice standard. The importance of the information is measured by the significance the reasonable person places upon it to go ahead with treatment. The main weakness of this approach is that it has been harder to use in practice.

The vast majority of patients with mental health problems are treated informally in that they agree to treatment and are willing to remain in hospital. Those treated informally have the right to refuse treatment and cannot be detained in hospital against their will. However, there are a number of patients with mental illness who lack the capacity to make an informed or rational decision. Here, we see paternalistic beneficence superseding autonomy; examples include taking action such as detaining the individual in hospital or giving treatment such as medication to prevent individuals harming themselves or others.

An individual being treated for a mental illness does not necessarily lack the capacity to make important and difficult decisions. The activity box asks you to consider the barriers to gaining informed consent and the scenario that follows looks at the issue of administering medication by concealment.

Activity 5.10   *Communication*

Apart from being under duress, what other barriers exist in gaining informed consent from a patient? Make a list of possible barriers, and also think of ways in which a nurse can overcome them.

An outline answer to this activity is given at the end of the chapter.

Scenario

You are caring for a 38-year-old man who is suffering from severe depression; he has made a number of recent attempts on his life. The patient sees no point in anything that is being done and is refusing to take medication as he believes there is nothing that can help him. You observe that your mentor is concealing anti-depressant medication in the patient's food. What are the ethical issues that arise from this situation and what guidance is there from your professional body, the NMC?

The concealment of medication is a complex issue; it can be acceptable in certain situations if it is considered in the best interests of the patient, such as preventing death. Here we see another example of paternalistic beneficence taking priority over patient autonomy. The NMC provides guidelines on the covert administration of medicine; for full details see the NMC website **www.nmc-uk.org**. Most clinical settings will have their own written policy on this matter. Some of the important points to consider are an assessment of the patient's mental capacity, their mental state and their best interests. This is not a decision to be taken by an individual; the issue needs wide discussion involving all of the mental health team in consultation with the patient's relatives.

Negligence

The cost of meeting claims for medical negligence has shown a steady increase since records have been kept. In 2010 the figure rose to £786,992,000 from £633,325,000 in 2008 (NHSLA (NHS Litigation Authority), 2010). In this section we will look at the law of negligence; this is an area of civil law, called tort law, which is concerned with the quality of relationship between individuals. Unlike in criminal law the wrong is committed against the individual rather than society, so the main functions of tort law are to provide compensation to the victim and to ensure that practitioners in future produce a high standard of work. Tort law seeks to establish a basic standard practice that should be expected as a minimum. Most of the cases that seek compensation will be heard in a civil court where, as mentioned earlier, it is easier to establish liability than in a criminal court (see Table 5.1 on page 73).

To establish if negligence has occurred and if compensation should be awarded, a number of elements must be established.

1. Is there a duty of care? In other words, does the nurse have a duty to care for this individual? Is it likely that an act or omission on the part of the nurse could result in harm to the individual? It is considered that a nurse owes a duty of care to those they are looking after.
2. Was there a breach in the duty of care? For example, was there a lack of care? Did the care fail to meet the expected standards?
3. Did this breach of the duty of care result in reasonably foreseeable harm?
4. Did harm occur, such as economic loss, injury to or the death of an individual?
   (Dimond, 2008)

In determining if negligence has occurred, the courts have to establish whether the act or omission of the nurse is a breach of their duty of care.

Vicarious liability

While the cause of negligence may be a failure on the part of the nurse, in practice legal action is taken against the nurse's employer, as few nurses would be able to bear the costs of such claims. Under the NHS Indemnity Scheme the employee is covered in cases of negligence, and this is known as vicarious liability.

Vicarious liability is the responsibility of one person for the actions of another because of their relationship, in this case a relationship of employment. So the **plaintiff** will take action against the hospital authority or, in the case of a private hospital, the company that owns the hospital. Once damages are awarded to the plaintiff, the employer can in theory sue the clinician responsible, but in practice this rarely occurs. For a fuller explanation of this area and of the Indemnity Scheme, see the NHS Litigation Authority website (NHSLA, nd).

Main legislation

In this section of the chapter we will identify some of the main legislation that needs to be considered in caring for those with mental health issues.

Human Rights Act 1998

The Human Rights Act 1998 came into effect on 2 October 2000 and requires any new legislation to comply with the European Convention on Human Rights and Fundamental

Freedoms (1950). The Act contains a number of rights and freedoms that apply to everyone in the UK. These include the right to life, liberty and security; a fair trial; respect for private and family life; marry; freedom of thought, conscience and religion; freedom of expression; freedom of assembly and association; prohibition of torture; prohibition of slavery and forced labour; no punishment without law; prohibition of discrimination.

The Human Rights Act is of particular importance for those caring for the mentally ill as the mentally ill will often find themselves the victims of stigmas and discrimination (Royal College of Psychiatry, 2008). As the mental health legislation gives those who care for the mentally ill powers to detain patients and treat them without agreement, it is important that clinicians are aware of the law and the responsibility that this entails. The case of Carol Savage and the successful legal action taken by her parents highlight this responsibility. Carol Savage was a 49-year-old woman who committed suicide; her parents successfully sued South Essex Partnership NHS Foundation Trust for breaching their daughter's human rights by not maintaining up-to-date documentation and failing to provide an appropriate level of observation – so by failing to maintain appropriate standards of care you can breach an individual's human rights.

One way to avoid an abuse of an individual's human rights is to adopt a human rights approach. Curtice and Exworthy (2009) propose the use of the FREDA principles where all interactions with patients are governed by fairness, respect, equality, dignity and autonomy. They further propose that all policies and procedures should reflect these principles. While the NMC Code (2008a) already expects that nurses' actions will be governed by these principles, nurses are best placed to identify those individuals who are most vulnerable, and to take steps to help them and their families to become empowered about their human rights.

Students wishing further information on using a human rights approach are advised to go to: **www.nhsemployers.org/Aboutus/Publications/Documents/NHSE_briefing69_180110.pdf**.

The Mental Health Acts 1983 and 2007

While 95 per cent of the people being treated for a mental illness will be treated informally (NHS ICHSC, 2010), as explained earlier they have the right to discharge themselves from hospital and refuse treatment, should they wish. However, due to the nature of mental illness, a number of these patients may be at risk from the community or indeed be a risk to the community or to themselves. As a result, this legislation allows an individual with a mental illness to be legally detained in a mental health care setting. The latest statistics show that there were 42,479 detentions in the period 2009–10, which was the largest increase in three years (NHS ICHSC, 2010). Working in a mental health environment may also bring you into contact with patients who have been referred to hospital by the criminal justice system under the Mental Health Act 2007, sections 45A and 47, for assessment and treatment. Students requiring information in this area should consult The NHS Information Centre for Health and Social Care at **www.ic.nhs.uk**.

While providing a legal framework for the detention of those with mental illness, the Mental Health Act 2007 also provides protection for the mentally ill from a society that can at times be hostile, and it has provision to curb overzealous interventions by the medical profession. A patient may have confided in you that they do not wish to receive a treatment or activity, or that they do not agree with the plan of their care but lack confidence in their own judgement and perceptions. As a mental health nurse you are bound by the NMC Code to *act as an advocate for those in your care* (NMC, 2008a, Section 4) and to *listen to the people in your care and respond to their concerns and preferences* (NMC, 2008a, Section 8). Here, you could represent the patient views and feelings on this matter at handovers and multidisciplinary team meetings. Further, you could support the patient by informing them of their rights under the Mental Health Act and telling them where to obtain information, also pointing out what external advocacy support is available. Detailed information on the advocacy support is available in the section on advocacy later in this chapter (on page 90).

The most current legislation on caring for the mentally ill is the Mental Health Act (MHA) 2007 which amended the Mental Health Act 1983. A brief overview follows; for a more in-depth understanding students should consult some of the further reading suggestions at the end of this chapter.

The Mental Health Act 2007 is arranged in various sections that allow for compulsory detention. The main sections you may encounter are Sections 2, 3, 4 and Section 136 (see Table 5.3). It is

Section	Time	Rationale
2	28 days	Assessment
3	6 months	Assessment and treatment
4	72 hours	Emergency admission
5(2)	72 hours	Doctors' holding power not renewable
5(4)	6 hours	Nurses' holding power not renewable.
17A	6 months	Community Treatment order
36	28 days to 12 weeks	Remand of accused person to hospital for treatment; can only be issued by a Crown Court
37	6 months	Issued by the Crown Court for convicted offenders who are suffering from a mental disorder
38	12 weeks	Interim hospital order
45A	Without limit of time	Issued by a Crown Court where a prison sentence is combined with a requirement for treatment
47		Transfer from prison plus restrictions
136	72 hours	A police officer can take a person whom they believe to be suffering from a mental disorder to a place of safety

Table 5.3: The main sections of the Mental Health Act 2007

important to remember that while only Section 3 allows for compulsory treatment, there are a number of emergency situations where treatment can be given under Part IV of the Mental Health Act 1983 without consent if a patient is detained under any of the following sections: 2, 3, 4, 36, 37, 38, 45A, 47.

Before any individual can be compulsorily detained, a medical recommendation and an application have to be completed, the exception being Section 136, which allows a police officer to remove an individual to a 'place of safety' if they believe the individual is suffering from a mental illness. A medical recommendation for Sections 2 or 3 requires two medical recommendations, in which one of the doctors would have to have attended an approved course within the last twelve months to meet the criteria for Section 12 of the MHA. In the case of Section 4, which is for an emergency admission for assessment for a period of 72 hours, only one medical recommendation is required. The application is normally made by an Approved Mental Health Professional (AMHP); while the nearest relative can make an application, this is rarely the case. Whereas prior to the MHA 2007 only Approved Social Workers (ASWs) could complete the application, now the function can be carried out by nurses, occupational therapists and psychologists once they have undergone the necessary training to become an AMHP.

A feature unique to mental health nursing is the use of holding powers Section 5(4). This allows a mental health nurse to detain a patient for up to six hours and should only be used as a temporary response in a crisis situation until a doctor can arrive on the scene. The most recent evidence shows that there were 1,579 occasions a year where this holding power is used by mental health nurses (NHS ICHSC, 2010).

To access the Mental Health Acts go to: **www.legislation.gov.uk**.

The Data Protection Act 1998

The Data Protection Act 1998 is a large and complex piece of legislation; it is the main legislation for governing the protection of personal data, and it has brought us into line with the existing legislation of the European Union. The Act concerns anyone who handles and stores personal information about individuals and places a number of legal obligations on individuals and organisations for the protection of this information; for example, you can only collect information that you need for a specific purpose. However, as we carry out holistic assessments of mental health patients, the range of information we gather can be quite broad.

It is permissible within the Act to place a marker – called a violent warning marker – on an individual's file if they pose or possibly pose a risk to staff. Care should be taken in applying these markers: the level of risk has to be established using objective criteria, and the type of violent behaviour that previously occurred has to be identified. The patient has to be informed of these actions, and they must be assessed regularly to see if a violent warning marker is still justified.

Mental Capacity Act 2005

The NMC Code Number 16 specifies that all nurses *must be aware of the legislation regarding mental capacity, ensuring that people who lack capacity remain at the centre of decision making and are fully safeguarded* (NMC, 2008a). A study by Grisso and Applebaum (1995) showed that nearly 50 per cent of patients with schizophrenia retained their capacity to make an informed decision. Further, Raymont et al. (2004) found that in general hospital populations, even after including those with gross cognitive impairment, only up to 31 per cent of in-patients lacked capacity. In the past, decisions about the care of patients without the capacity to make their own decisions would be dealt with under the common law of necessity; now such decisions are taken in keeping with the framework provided by the Mental Capacity Act.

The Mental Capacity Act 2005 came into effect in 2007. It states that *for the purpose of this Act a person lacks capacity in relation to a matter if at the material time he is unable to make a decision for himself in relation to the matter because of an impairment of, or a disturbance in the functioning of, the mind or brain.* It goes on to add that it *does not matter whether the impairment or disturbance is permanent or temporary* (DH, 2005). The main principles of the Act are as follows.

- A presumption of capacity – every adult has the right to make his or her own decisions and must be assumed to have capacity to do so unless it is proved otherwise.
- Individuals being supported to make their own decisions – a person must be given all practicable help before anyone treats them as not being able to make their own decisions.
- Unwise decisions – just because an individual makes what might be seen as an unwise decision, they should not be treated as lacking capacity to make that decision.
- Best interests – an act done or decision made under the Act for or on behalf of a person who lacks capacity must be done in their best interests.
- Least restrictive option – anything done for or on behalf of a person who lacks capacity should be the least restrictive of their basic rights and freedoms.

In order for clinicians to assess if an individual has the capacity to make decisions about their care, they must satisfy the following criteria (Section 3 of the Act). They must be able to understand the information relevant to the decision; retain that information; use or weigh that information as part of the process of making the decision; communicate their decision (whether by talking, using sign language or any other means). If an individual is unable to meet all of these criteria, the clinician is able to make a decision in their best interests. To assist in deciding what is in the best interests of an individual, Section 4 of the Act includes a best interests checklist of items that should be taken into account.

- Likelihood that the individual will regain their capacity at a later date.
- Participation by the individual in the decision making as far as possible.
- The person's past and present wishes.
- The beliefs and values of the patient.
- The views of people appointed to speak for the patient.
- The views of anyone who has been granted power of attorney for the patient.
- Advance decisions made by the patient about the care they would be willing to receive when they had capacity.
- Decisions not to be based on the person's age or appearance, or aspect of their behaviour.

Making decisions on behalf of others is a difficult area; however, there are a number of guidelines for those in the clinical environment (see 'Useful websites' at the end of the chapter).

The Equality Act 2010

As a mental health nurse you are expected to provide care that does not discriminate in any way against those in your care. The main aim of the Equality Act is to bring together and clarify nine major laws on equality and numerous other pieces of legislation that attempt to address discrimination in Great Britain (Northern Ireland is not included). It replaces legislation such as the Equal Pay Act 1970, Sex Discrimination Act 1975, Race Relations Act 1976, and the Disability Discrimination Act 1995, so for the first time there is now a single Act that covers discrimination in areas such, race, age, sexuality and disability. The Act places new duties upon public bodies such as councils, educational providers and hospitals to consider how they can make sure that people are not at a disadvantage because of disability or social background. Further, all public bodies must treat people equally and fairly regardless of their background. The Act offers new protection for people who are looking after someone – such as parents caring for a disabled son or daughter – from being treated unfairly. For example, employers cannot refuse to employ a person who is caring for a disabled relative because they think they will have to take time off work. Education providers may have to provide special equipment such as recording equipment or ensure access to facilities to those who are physically impaired. For further information on this area, see 'Useful websites' at the end of the chapter.

Safeguards

In this last section we will identify some of the many measures in place to safeguard those in care with mental health problems. The nature of mental illness and the complexity of the care and treatment of the mentally ill, coupled with the power imbalance that is often a feature of the relationship between patients and care providers, are such that there needs to be in place a number of safeguards to protect patients. In 2000 the Department of Health published *No secrets* (DH, 2000), which provided guidance on protecting vulnerable adults from abuse. It defined a vulnerable adult as a person:

> *who is or may be in need of community care services by reason of mental or other disability, age or illness* **and** *who is or may be unable to take care of him or herself, **or** unable to protect him or herself against harm or exploitation.*

In March 2011 the Department of Health provided further guidance with the publication of *Safeguarding adults* (DH, 2011b); it identifies six principles that can provide a foundation for good practice.

- Empowerment: presumption of person-led decisions and consent.
- Protection: support and representation for those in greatest need.
- Prevention: prevention of harm as a primary objective.
- Proportionality: proportionality and least intrusive response appropriate to the risk presented.
- Partnerships: local solutions through services working with their communities.
- Accountability: accountability and transparency in delivering safeguarding.

There is a wide range of measures in place to protect the patient. First, individuals wishing to become nurses will have to be checked to see if they have a criminal record (CRB check) and, if so, whether their offences are such that they may prove a risk to vulnerable patients. Further, nurses are registered by a professional body – the NMC – which provides professional standards and a code of conduct. A nurse whose level of practice is deemed unsafe will be removed from the register and thereafter will be unable to practise as a nurse. The Code requires a nurse to obtain a patient's consent before carrying out any procedures. It also obligates the nurse to fully involve the patient in decisions about their care, by inviting questions, explaining procedures and pointing out the risks so that informed consent may be obtained.

Advocacy

Action for Advocacy (2002) defines advocacy as *taking action to help people say what they want, secure their rights, represent their interests and obtain services they need.* It takes many forms: as a nurse you will have to support patients in expressing their views or to speak on their behalf. While we are obligated to speak up on behalf of those in our care, some writers, such as Jugessur and Iles (2009) in a review of nurse advocacy, have pointed out that this role may give rise to conflict between service users, medical staff and employers, and for this reason they question how effective nurses can be in this role. There are also local advocacy groups who will visit clinical areas and hold regular meetings at which patients can seek help, often from people who have themselves recovered from mental health problems, and there are independent advocates such as Independent Mental Health Advocates (IMHAs) and Independent Mental Capacity Advocates (IMCAs) (see 'Useful websites' at the end of the chapter).

Living wills and advance health directives

Under the Mental Capacity Act 2005 advance health directives are now legally enforceable. An individual can therefore now specify in advance the care and treatment they would wish to receive (or not) should they ever be unable to express their wishes (see 'Useful websites' for more information). The decisions that individuals make regarding their future care and treatment are legally binding if the advance directive meets the following requirements.

- The person making the directive was 18 or older when it was made, and had the necessary mental capacity.
- It specifies, in lay terms if necessary, the specific treatment to be refused and the particular circumstances in which the refusal is to apply.
- The person making the directive has not withdrawn the decision at a time when they had the capacity to do so.
- The person making the directive has not appointed, after the directive was made, an attorney to make the specified decision.
- The person making the directive has not done anything clearly inconsistent with the directive remaining a fixed decision.

Patients' rights

There are a number of ways in which a patient or relative can complain about the quality of treatment that has been given. Under the Hospital Complaints Procedure Act 1985 a patient or a relative of a patient may submit a written complaint and the complaint will be investigated by the complaints officer of the Trust in question. The complainant will receive an acknowledgement of the complaint within three working days of the date on which the complaint was made. Further, a copy of the complaint will be forwarded to all parties named in the complaint. Individuals making a complaint can receive support from the Independent Complaints Advocacy Service (ICAS), which offers a free, independent and confidential service. Further information on the ICAS is available at **www.pohwer.net**. The Department of Health produces a large number leaflets that are only available via the web – see 'Useful websites' at the end of the chapter.

The Care Quality Commission

The Care Quality Commission (CQC) is responsible for the licensing and monitoring of care services provided by NHS, local authorities and voluntary agencies to make sure that care meets an acceptable level. In March 2010, in order to measure the quality of care, the CQC produced Essential Standards of Quality and Safety, and from October 2010 these standards became legally binding upon all health and social care services.

- You can expect to be involved and told what is happening at every stage of your care.
- You can expect care, treatment and support that meet your needs.
- You can expect to be safe.
- You can expect to be cared for by qualified staff.
- You can expect your care provider to constantly check the quality of its services.

The CQC also provides Mental Health Act Commissioners who visit service users detained in hospital or on Community Treatment Orders (CTOs). The Mental Health Commissioners protect the rights of detained service users by visiting the clinical areas; these visits can be unannounced, that is, no warning is given of their coming. MHA Commissioners provide further safeguards to good practice by listening to the concerns of patients and raising their concerns with senior staff, assisting in the writing of letters or complaints. They also monitor the quality of care by checking the documentation and the publishing of reports on clinical areas.

Deprivation of Liberty (Bournewood) Safeguards

In 2008 the Mental Capacity Act 2005 was amended with the introduction of Deprivation of Liberty Safeguards (Code of Practice) in April 2009 (see 'Useful websites' at the end of the chapter).

Chapter summary

This chapter explored the subject of ethics, how we develop our values and how they impact upon our decision making. We identified the four ethical principles of autonomy, beneficence, non-maleficence and justice, and considered how to apply these principles in clinical practice. In our discussion on the legal system an overview of the judicial system works was given, the types of law and how they relate to nursing. The role and function of the NMC was outlined. The legal aspects of nursing were explored with reference to areas such as consent and negligence, and the main areas of legislation identified and discussed. Lastly, this chapter focused on the safeguarding of service users and the measures that are available such as advocacy, patients' rights, living wills and the various agencies involved in this work.

Activities: brief outline answers

Activity 5.3: Critical thinking (page 73)

This case presents us with a number of safeguarding issues that calls for input from a wide range of professionals. The CAMHS team needs to explain the risks that this individual is exposing herself to. Further, as she is having unprotected sex there is a risk of sexually transmitted diseases and pregnancy. A referral to family planning services should be arranged where advice on contraception could be given. As she is refusing to allow her parents to be informed, contraception could given to this girl under the Fraser guidelines, if she has understood the advice given, if staff have failed to persuade her to inform her parents and if she is most likely going to continue to have sex. There are also child protection issues here. As she is having sex with men who are older than her, there is a possibility that she is being abused; social services should be involved and possibly the police.

Activity 5.4: Critical thinking (page 74)

This is a clear breach of the Code in a number of areas. The nursing staff failed to provide a high standard of care. Ann delegated the care to junior staff, and her level of supervision of her staff was inadequate. The staff failed to respect the patient or to show consideration for her injuries. They also failed to provide care that was best practice and to keep accurate records. The nursing staff would be suspended by their employers, the Trust, while there was an investigation. If the verdict found that gross misconduct had occurred, the staff in question could be dismissed, and the case would then be referred to the NMC as a fitness for practice issue. The NMC could place an interim suspension order preventing the staff in question from working while there were concerns about their level of practice. In view of the level of misconduct, the outcome of the NMC investigation could result in the staff being struck off the register. Lastly, the relatives could take legal action against the Trust, claiming that negligence had occurred.

Activity 5.5: Reflection (page 74)

Some of you may have felt that the function of the NMC is to promote and develop the profession of nursing. However, in reading this chapter you have no doubt identified that the main function of the NMC is to safeguard the public while they are in the care of nurses. This may surprise you, but as we have seen over this chapter, there are an increasing number of complaints being made about the quality of care given by some nurses.

Activity 5.6: Reflection (page 75)

You may have included doctors, lawyers, priests, nurses and teachers. But what is it that they all share? It is true that they all have lengthy periods of training but they do not share the same level of status or indeed financial reward. Arguably, some footballers have more prestige, but is being a footballer a profession (although the phrase 'professional foul' is commonly used)? We hear the phrases 'being professional' and 'acting professionally'; often these refer to your appearance at work or how you conduct yourself. While the last points have their place, most of us would rather be treated by an effective but unconventional clinician than by a conventional but ineffective one. You might have identified the following as some of the reasons that nursing is a profession: an expectation with regard to moral behaviour, the need to show integrity, and putting the needs of your clients or the people in your charge before your own needs.

Activity 5.7: Reflection (page 76)

The NMC registers all nurses and midwives, and ensures that they are properly qualified and competent to work in the UK. It sets the standards of education, training and conduct that nurses and midwives need to deliver high-quality health care consistently throughout their careers. It ensures that nurses and midwives keep their skills and knowledge up to date and uphold the standards of their professional code. It ensures that midwives are safe to practise by setting rules for their practice and supervision. It has fair processes to investigate allegations made against nurses and midwives who may not have followed the Code (NMC, 2010a).

Activity 5.9: Communication (page 82)

Other examples are:

- I will have to inform the consultant that you are not being cooperative.
- If you don't take your medication the consultant will be very unhappy.
- You don't want what happened to . . . to happen to you.
- What you are doing could prolong your illness.
- I've explained all this to you already!

Activity 5.10: Communication (page 83)

Barriers to gaining consent.

- Sensory impairment.
- Poor interpersonal skills on the part of the nurse.
- Lacking knowledge of the treatment.
- Patient fails to engage due to bad experience of past treatment.
- Patient lacking confidence to ask questions.
- Not spending enough time to explain treatment.

Measures to overcome barriers in gaining informed consent.

- Take time in explaining procedures and treatment.
- Give time for the individual to make their decision.
- Consider measures to overcome sensory problems such as facing and looking at the individual when speaking to them.
- Invite questions.
- Clarify if the individual understands the procedure or what is expected of them.
- Allow the individual to exercise personal preferences where possible.
- Provide information in a manner that can be understood by the individual, e.g. avoid jargon.
- Be truthful; don't make exaggerated claims; if you don't know the answer to the question asked, then say so.

Further reading

Brown, R (2009) *The approved mental health professional's guide to mental health law*, 2nd edition. Exeter: Learning Matters.

Dimond, B (2008) *Legal aspects of nursing*, 5th edition. Harlow: Pearson.

Thompson, I, Melia, K, Boyd, K and Horsburgh, D (2006) *Nursing ethics*, 5th edition. Oxford: Churchill Livingstone.

South London and Maudsley NHS Foundation Trust (2010) *The Maze: guide to the Mental Health Act 2007*. London: South London and Maudsley NHS Foundation Trust.

Useful websites

www.cqc.org.uk

Further information on the Care Quality Commission and on the guide it published in October 2010.

www.pohwer.net

Further information on the IMHA or IMCA can be obtained on this website, which is the POhWER *Advocacy, making your voice heard* website.

www.direct.gov.uk

www.patient.co.uk

More information on living wills is available on these websites.

www.direct.gov.uk

On this website you will find guidance material on making decisions on behalf of others.

www.equalities.gov.uk

Advice on disability and discrimination is given here.

www.dh.gov.uk

Go to this website for a fuller understanding of *Safeguarding adults*.

www.dh.gov.uk/en/Publicationsandstatistics/Publications/PublicationsPolicyAndGuidance /DH_089275

www.adviceguide.org.uk

www.patients-association.com

www.mind.org.uk

These websites all give information on patients' rights.

www.dhov.uk/en/Publicationsandstatistics/Publications/PublicationsPolicyAndGuidance /DH_085476

This is the web link for the Deprivation of Liberty Safeguards (Code of Practice).

Chapter 6
Communicating and relating

Reuben Pearce

NMC Standards for Pre-registration Nursing Education

This chapter will address the following competencies:

Domain 1: Professional values

2. All nurses must practise in a holistic, non-judgmental, caring and sensitive manner that avoids assumptions, supports social inclusion; recognises and respects individual choice; and acknowledges diversity. Where necessary, they must challenge inequality, discrimination and exclusion from access to care.

Domain 2: Communication and interpersonal skills

1. All nurses must build partnerships and therapeutic relationships through safe, effective and non-discriminatory communication. They must take account of individual differences, capabilities and needs.

2. All nurses must use a range of communication skills and technologies to support person-centred care and enhance quality and safety. They must ensure people receive all the information they need in a language and manner that allows them to make informed choices and share decision making. They must recognise when language interpretation or other communication support is needed and know how to obtain it.

3. All nurses must use the full range of communication methods, including verbal, non-verbal and written, to acquire, interpret and record their knowledge and understanding of people's needs. They must be aware of their own values and beliefs and the impact this may have on their communication with others. They must take account of the many different ways in which people communicate and how these may be influenced by ill health, disability and other factors, and be able to recognise and respond effectively when a person finds it hard to communicate.

4. All nurses must recognise when people are anxious or in distress and respond effectively, using therapeutic principles, to promote their well-being, manage personal safety and resolve conflict. They must use effective communication strategies and negotiation techniques to achieve best outcomes, respecting the dignity and human rights of all concerned. They must know when to consult a third party and how to make referrals for advocacy, mediation or arbitration.

5. All nurses must use therapeutic principles to engage, maintain and, where appropriate, disengage from professional caring relationships, and must always respect professional boundaries.

continued overleaf . . .

continued . . .

6. All nurses must take every opportunity to encourage health-promoting behaviour through education, role modelling and effective communication.

7. All nurses must maintain accurate, clear and complete records, including the use of electronic formats, using appropriate and plain language.

8. All nurses must respect individual rights to confidentiality and keep information secure and confidential in accordance with the law and relevant ethical and regulatory frameworks, taking account of local protocols. They must also actively share personal information with others when the interests of safety and protection override the need for confidentiality.

Domain 3: Nursing practice and decision-making

4. All nurses must ascertain and respond to the physical, social and psychological needs of people, groups and communities. They must then plan, deliver and evaluate safe, competent, person-centred care in partnership with them, paying special attention to changing health needs during different life stages, including progressive illness and death, loss and bereavement.

7. All nurses must be able to recognise and interpret signs of normal and deteriorating mental and physical health and respond promptly to maintain or improve the health and comfort of the service user, acting to keep them and others safe.

Domain 4: Leadership, management and team working

4. All nurses must be self-aware and recognise how their own values, principles and assumptions may affect their practice. They must maintain their own personal and professional development, learning from experience, through supervision, feedback, reflection and evaluation.

NMC Essential Skills Clusters

Cluster: Care, compassion and communication

1. As partners in the care process, people can trust a newly registered graduate nurse to provide collaborative care based on the highest standards, knowledge and competence.

2. People can trust the newly registered graduate nurse to engage in person centred care empowering people to make choices about how their needs are met when they are unable to meet them for themselves.

3. People can trust the newly registered graduate nurse to respect them as individuals and strive to help them to preserve their dignity at all times.

4. People can trust a newly qualified graduate nurse to engage with them and their family or carers within their cultural environments in an acceptant and anti-discriminatory manner free from harassment and exploitation.

5. People can trust the newly registered graduate nurse to engage with them in a warm, sensitive and compassionate way.

continued overleaf . . .

continued . . .

6. People can trust the newly registered graduate nurse to engage therapeutically and actively listen to their needs and concerns, responding using skills that are helpful, providing information that is clear, accurate, meaningful and free from jargon.

Cluster: Organisational aspects of care

9. People can trust the newly registered graduate nurse to treat them as partners and work with them to make a holistic and systematic assessment of their needs; to develop a personalised plan that is based on mutual understanding and respect for their individual situation promoting health and well-being, minimising risk of harm and promoting their safety at all times.

Chapter aims

By the end of this chapter, you should be able to:

* consider how you interact with other people;
* explore the therapeutic relationship;
* discuss psychological approaches to relating with others;
* highlight and discuss key skills for effective communication;
* examine common barriers to effective communication;
* consider managing difficult situations and dealing with conflict.

Introduction

Throughout this chapter you will explore and discuss the importance of professional communication and how it can help nurses develop therapeutic alliances when relating with people who might be experiencing mental distress. Everybody has to communicate with people through their daily activities in order to function as human beings in society. Although this book is applied in the mental health context, the skills discussed in this chapter can be applied across the board both personally and professionally. Communicating is vital for people to survive in their activities of daily living and so it is a crucial part of your role as a health care professional. Being able to communicate and relate to people and their unique experience of mental distress is vital for meaningful and effective nursing intervention.

Activity 6.1   *Reflection*

Consider for a moment a time when you may have communicated a message without realising it at the time. For example, have you ever decided that you want to spend an evening in your room on your own, maybe watching TV?

• What might this demonstrate to the people you live with?
• How might they perceive your actions?
• Could their perception of what you are communicating be different from what you are in reality thinking?

As this activity is based on your own experiences, there is no outline answer at the end of the chapter.

Can you see how people communicate unconsciously even when they are not aware that what they are doing is conveying a message?

Now consider another example, such as one of those awkward moments that you might find yourself in where you have to speak to somebody whom you really do not want to speak with. Despite doing your best to have a friendly chat, your body language can reveal your true feelings to the other person without you realising.

Activity 6.2   *Reflection*

Reflect upon a time when you have come away from speaking to somebody feeling angry or negative.

• Was there something about the person's attitude?
• How were you feeling at the time in the moments just prior to the interaction?
• Were you already feeling worried and stressed about something else?

As this activity is based on your own experiences, there is no outline answer at the end of the chapter.

It is likely that once you have given some thought to Activity 6.2 you will have realised that everybody will have irritated somebody unconsciously by something that they have said or through a look on their face; it happens on many occasions throughout people's day-to-day lives. As already mentioned, the skills discussed in this chapter will have relevance to your everyday life, both personally and professionally as a nurse.

When working with people who are mentally distressed, the skills of communicating and relating take arguably the most crucial role in engaging an individual to the point that collaborative assessment and helping can occur (Bowers et al., 2009). If there is poor communication from the start, this can prevent the nurse from getting as far as assessing or helping that person. In fact, poor communication alongside lack of self-awareness can even lead to gross misinterpretation of someone's behaviour (McCabe and Timmins, 2006). For example, you may have a patient who seems to be behaving in an aggressive manner. The anger may have been triggered by a nurse's lack of interest demonstrated in their body language and general attitude. The nurse, unaware of their own attitude and its impact on the situation, records in their nursing report that the patient was uncooperative, agitated and angry. You may agree that this seems very unfair and that the situation could have been completely avoided if the nurse had demonstrated appropriate communication skills.

It is through adopting excellent communication skills that positive relationships with patients and their carers can be developed and difficult situations avoided. Through striking up a strong therapeutic relationship with people experiencing mental distress, nurses can better identify their individual needs (Thurgood, 2009). As a nurse your awareness of how you interact and relate should not be restricted to the patient but should also include their relatives, friends and carers. Through building therapeutic alliances inclusive of friends, families and carers, nurses can provide a more holistic and person-centred package of care (Firn, 2008). Take a moment to consider how we communicate both verbally and non-verbally. Think of some examples of these that you might use in practice.

The therapeutic relationship

In 1952 Hildegard Peplau introduced the idea of the therapeutic relationship as a *human connection that heals*. Peplau (1988) has highlighted how the interpersonal work that nurses do makes a unique contribution to health care. The therapeutic relationship can be viewed as an alliance that is formed between a nurse, a patient and their family and/or carers for a certain period of time. The aim of the relationship will be to achieve certain goals related to promoting the health and well-being of the patient. The relationship will have stages that include a beginning, a middle and an end.

> **Theory summary: Peplau's stages of the nurse–patient relationship (Peplau, 1988)**
>
> 1. Orientation phase.
> 2. Working phase (active intervention).
>   - Identification.
>   - Exploitation.
> 3. Termination/resolution phase.

Peplau (1988) suggested that the **orientation phase** can set the scene for the rest of the relationship and is often part of the initial assessment. This can be seen as the stage in which the issues are identified in a collaborative manner. Once issues are identified, the relationship is ready to move on to the working phase that has two components: identification and exploitation.

The **identification** part of the phase is the clarification between the nurse and patient on ideas and expectations from intervention. This can be seen as the care planning stage. The **exploitation** component is about making as much use as possible of the patient's own personal strengths and resources to promote empowerment. You can consider the exploitation component as the doing stage.

The final stage of the relationship, known as the **termination** or **resolution phase**, is when the progress of the intervention is evaluated to see if the issues originally identified have been resolved or improved.

The therapeutic relationship can only be as good as the sum of these parts and so can easily deteriorate at any of the phases mentioned above. If you do not strike up a good rapport in the orientation stage, then you will have trouble in the working phase, if you manage to get there at all. Likewise, if you are unable to get past a superficial politeness in the orientation phase you may not reach the real issues in the working phase. When you come to the termination phase and fail to evaluate and acknowledge the relationship coming to its end you can jeopardise all the work that has gone in previously and the patient may not want to engage in the future because they have no trust in the system (Peplau, 1988; Underman Boggs, 2007a).

It is probably idealistic to believe that your interactions will run smoothly through each of these stages. You may find yourself returning to the first two phases at a point when you hoped you might be at phase three, and this is due to the complex nature of mental distress. Through remaining flexible and being able to adapt to the patient's presentation you maintain a patient-centred approach to care. It is important to remember that patients do not necessarily live in isolation and will generally belong to a wider system; they live as part of a family, and have friends and other social and environmental networks (Weinstein, 2008). Traditionally, these fundamental components of a person's sense of well-being have not been taken into account in health-care settings. Gaining consent and collaborating with families and/or carers can aid the recovery process through addressing care needs more holistically (Simpson and Brennan, 2009).

Establishing a working understanding of psychological theory and reflective practice that underpins communicating and relating can help you in working through these stages, so this will be discussed in the next part of the chapter.

Self-awareness through reflective practice

In order to be effective, professional skilled communicators you need to develop your level of self-awareness through reflective practice. Let us take a look at applying Kolb's experiential cycle (Kolb, 1984) to demonstrate how people learn from experience (see Figure 6.1). Kolb claims that 'learning' is done through the process of a cycle. This cycle calls people to observe and reflect on an experience, then to conceptualise abstract theories and then to experiment with what they have learned in their future practice (Jasper, 2003). It can be relevant to apply Kolb's model to your role as a nurse to enable you to think critically about your interactions and the application

Concrete Experience
(doing/having an experience)

Active Experimentation
(planning/trying out what you have learned)

Reflective Observation
(reviewing/reflecting on the experience)

Abstract Conceptualisation
(concluding/learning from the experience)

Figure 6.1: Kolb's cycle of learning

Source: Kolb, 1984.

of nursing theory to practice. To aid the reflective process some understanding of psychological theories that explain a bit about human behaviour can help you in understanding yourself and others in the therapeutic relationship.

The psychodynamic approach

Sigmund Freud was the founder of psychoanalysis during the 1890s. This approach in counselling explores inner defence mechanisms, dreams, the unconscious and hidden meaning. Have you ever heard somebody mention the Freudian slip? Having touched upon unconscious communication at the beginning of the chapter and in light of this, it is worth considering some of Freud's ideas. Freud held the belief that the way we behave and interact as humans is unconsciously influenced by each of our past experiences, values and beliefs. He introduced the theory of transference and counter-transference as a means of explaining the dynamic in an interaction that can create certain feelings within us (Howard, 2010).

Transference is what happens when individuals unconsciously project feelings and attitudes towards others that are based on previous experiences or relationships (McCabe and Timmins, 2006). In your relationships as nurses with people who are experiencing emotional distress you might, for example, find yourself communicating with a person unconsciously about a past relationship or experience that is unrelated to the present situation. Talking to an older authoritative male nurse may arouse feelings of anger stemming from fear in a person who has unresolved issues relating to childhood physical and emotional abuse from their father.

Case study

Jimmy is a 25-year-old self-employed gardener; he is a patient in the A&E department following an accident at work that resulted in a possible fracture to his hand. Jimmy is highly anxious as he needs the use of his hand to be able to work, and he starts to become rather agitated towards Rachael, the nurse on duty. He tells her quite sharply that he has been waiting ages. This annoys Rachael and she tells Jimmy to be more polite or he won't get seen at all. Rachael feels really annoyed as she has already been spoken to badly today by two previous patients and also by her husband.

Rachael may be feeling less tolerant than usual because she has been shouted at earlier in the day, and so she speaks in quite a sharp way to the patient. Jimmy may feel rejected, and his feelings of worthlessness are unconsciously reinforced by the nurse.

Scenario

You are out for a home visit with a nurse who has been seeing a 54-year-old woman who suffers from very low mood. She is often very tearful, and it seems that there is very little that is positive in her life at the moment. The patient gets very upset and tearful about a falling-out she has had with a friend who had forgotten her birthday, and she also mentions that she is upset with the nurse who had forgotten to acknowledge that it was her birthday. The nurse internally feels irritated by the patient – she thinks to herself: 'What does she expect from me? I'm her nurse not her best friend. Does she not think I'm busy enough already?' The nurse is a little bit short in her response and says to the patient: 'Well, I am sorry but I have been very busy and I can't be remembering the birthday of everyone I see.' The nurse immediately feels very guilty, is extremely apologetic and offers to see the patient again the following day, when she would normally see her only once a week.

Activity 6.3   *Critical thinking*

* What do you think might be happening in this scenario?
* Do you think the nurse is going to help the patient by offering her the extra visit?
* Reflect upon situations in your own life. Have you ever encountered similar situations?

There is an outline answer at the end of the chapter.

Transference theory would suggest that the patient might not really have been angry with the nurse or even with her friend but was most likely angry with a parental figure who often forgot special days in her life. If a patient is in therapy, then the therapist might talk this through with a view to the patient gaining a better understanding of why they feel they way they do. The nurse in this situation felt guilty and started to feel the need to rescue the upset patient, slipping into the role of the absent parent. This was exacerbated by the nurse's own transference issues: the nurse felt stressed at how busy she was, which led to her feeling irritated by the patient. **Counter-transference** is our own emotional response (counter-reaction) to somebody else's transference and is likely to include our own transference issues. Counter-transference by nurses will often manifest as over-involvement and/or withdrawal. It is very easy when working with emotionally distressed people to become over-involved because of the need that the upset person brings out in us to help them. Now this is obviously not a bad thing; a desire to help people is what brings most people into the nursing profession in the first place, and if you do not want to help people then you are probably in the wrong profession. However, sometimes the reason you feel such a strong need to help people is because you have absorbed lots of their inner turmoil and have started to feel helpless yourself. Now this can lead you to satisfying your own need to feel better for helping them when actually you could be making them feel worse by disempowering them.

The other danger is that you get over-involved to a point where you feel completely saturated and burnt out with a patient. This can lead to you feeling as though you cannot continue to work with the patient and can result in reinforcing the patient's low self-esteem because they then feel rejected.

Recognising your responses to relationships through the use of reflection can raise your self-awareness so that you challenge the feelings and reconsider them. This is why in mental health nursing there is a great emphasis on **clinical supervision**. Clinical supervision gives a clinician regular protected time to reflect on practice with another clinician. The second clinician can take an objective look at the interactions and relationships of the person being supervised in order to maintain and build upon good practice and learn from difficulties encountered (RCN, 2003a).

The humanistic approach

Carl Rogers is famous for introducing the person-centred approach to interpersonal communication. He identified three main components of person-centred theory; these were warmth, empathy and genuineness (Rogers, 1959). Rogers believed that warmth was very important in the early stages of the therapeutic relationship in order to build rapport. According to Rogers, warmth is demonstrated through exhibiting **unconditional positive regard** towards other people. This is showing respect for a person as an individual through being non-judgemental. Empathy will be discussed in more detail later in the chapter; however, empathy demonstrates to the other person that we appreciate their experience for what it means to them. Integral to effective empathic skills is the ability to demonstrate genuineness, and this was a concept close to Rogers' heart. Genuineness may be achieved through disregarding your own views and feelings when working with a patient and accepting them as a unique individual, i.e. not looking just at the symptoms of an illness or a person's appearance, but looking at the whole person and their journey, leaving your own prejudices, values and beliefs to one side. You can also demonstrate genuineness through your behaviour being congruent. For example, you might say all the right things verbally but look somewhat disinterested non-verbally. In order to come across as genuine, your verbal and non-verbal behaviours should be aligned (Churchill, 2011).

Both Carl Rogers and another pioneer of human psychology named Abraham Maslow were from the humanistic school of psychology. Maslow (1999) felt that people have a set of needs that drive them, beginning with more basic needs such as those to survive and belong through to the need for self-esteem and ultimately **self-actualisation**. Self-actualisation may be seen simply as feeling great in all aspects of life. In order to get to this point a person needs to have achieved the basic survival needs right through to full self-esteem. Maslow developed a hierarchy of these needs to help with understanding of the concept (see Figure 6.2). He said that very few people ever get to self-actualisation, describing it as a journey rather than a goal. Maslow's theory can be helpful when working with people experiencing mental distress as through identifying their current state of need you are able to establish what level of intervention they might be ready for. The humanistic approach tends to lean towards considering people as a whole rather than as a set of components.

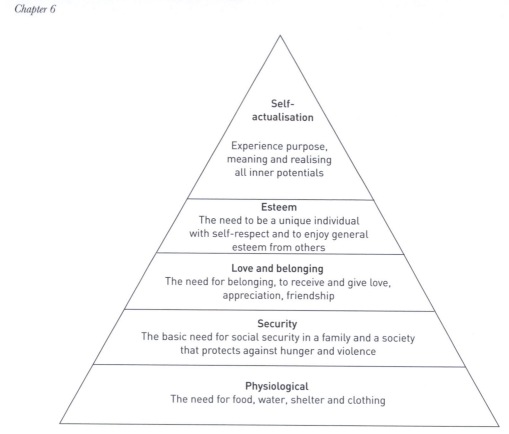

Figure 6.2: Maslow's hierarchy of needs

Core skills that can lead to effective therapeutic communication

First impressions count

The ability of a nurse to effectively use core communication skills such as listening, questioning, touch, paraphrasing and body language will directly influence the development of the trusting relationship. Building a good rapport will lay the foundations for the therapeutic relationship (Sin and Trenoweth, 2010). If you reflect on many of your own interactions, you can probably assume that you often make very quick decisions over whether you like someone or not, sometimes within seconds or minutes of meeting them. This demonstrates how much first impressions count, and it is therefore important that you work hard on those initial rapport building stages of your interactions with people who are mentally distressed (Sanders, 2003). When a person is mentally distressed, some basic communication skills that people value when they meet people for the first time can be lost – such as a warm smile and non-verbal acknowledgement. This may be due to personal anxiety about how to manage the situation. Setting the scene for an interaction is crucial when working with mental distress. Remembering to introduce yourself, your role and why you are there, offering a warm smile, offering eye contact and giving careful consideration to your opening statement can really make a difference to the success of the intervention. Remember to be reading for verbal/non-verbal communication cues as you enter the room to greet the person. 'How are you today?' with a big smile may not always be an appropriate greeting for somebody who is extremely depressed, agitated or angry and you could receive a curt response. In this case it may be more appropriate to start the consultation with an empathic statement (more on this later) such as 'I can see that you are very distressed – thanks for taking the time to see me.' You can also introduce yourself and verbalise your observation by saying 'I can see that you are very upset – I am here to see if there is something I can do to help you.'

Active listening

Excellent listening skills are absolutely key to successfully engaging people who are experiencing mental distress. A nurse who is demonstrating high-quality active listening skills can sometimes begin to help someone who is distressed feel better based on the use of those skills alone (Kagan and Evans, 1995). Active listening demonstrates to the distressed person that you can appreciate what their difficulties mean to them as an individual and can give the distressed person comfort because they get a sense of genuine concern and interest from the nurse (Chambers and Ryder, 2009). Active listening is more than just demonstrating patience and hearing. It involves a range of skills that can be developed by you as a nurse to add to your tool kit for communicating and relating. The following three key components to active listening can provide the mentally distressed patient with a safe emotional space to think and talk (McCabe and Timmins, 2006).

- Appropriate use of silence.
- Minimal verbal interruption.
- The demonstration of active listening through body language.

Active listening also provides the nurse with time to reflect and consider their verbal interaction, so that it is appropriate, constructive and person-centred. Silence can make you feel uncomfortable, and you might feel the need to fill the silence with words, which can often be unnecessary and be more about your uncomfortable feeling with the silence rather than about what the person experiencing distress is feeling (Stein-Parbury, 2005).

Activity 6.4   *Communication*

Have you ever considered your sitting position when talking to patients? Try sitting directly opposite a colleague with little distance between you. Now try sitting side by side and having a conversation. Now try a 90-degree angle.

- What position feels the least threatening?
- What position feels most personally disconnected?
- What sitting position would you feel most comfortable with?

An outline answer is given at the end of the chapter.

More non-verbal techniques that support active listening

As seen in Activity 6.4, through considering your seating position, so that it is not too opposing yet not too distant, you can demonstrate that you are ready to listen while putting the patient at ease. The aim can then be to maintain a relaxed 'open' body position, leaning slightly towards the patient and giving good eye contact throughout the interaction. (Remember not to over-compensate and stare someone out.) These non-verbal skills are known as **attending**. Attending is the physical demonstration that you are interested and ready to listen (Underman Boggs, 2007b). It is also important when working in, for example, a fast-paced A&E department to give the perception of time to the patient. You can both consciously and unconsciously give the impression that you are very busy, and the patient is then less likely to engage either through annoyance or through fear of being a burden.

There are verbal components to active listening and these include clarification, feedback and **summarising**. Summarising is repeating what someone else has said in your own words. In order to do this you need to have been listening carefully. Summarising demonstrates to the patient that you really have been listening and are interested in what they are saying. It also prevents misunderstandings and misinterpretation of information (provides clarification) and encourages communication that is open through feedback (Moss, 2008). You can view this as an opportunity to formulate your thoughts about what you have been told. Summarising can also highlight genuineness to the patient, as it is an open and non-judgemental technique (Rogers, 1959). Remember to make sure your body language is congruent with the words that you use. **Clarification** can be important and can be described as the skill of seeking clarification of your own understanding of the patient's experience – you might think of this as a way of checking with your patient that you understand them correctly and it plays an important role similar to and in conjunction with summarising.

The giving and receiving of **feedback** are also important skills to develop. It is only through receiving feedback that you may be able to see yourself as others see you. This can obviously be a bit frightening – you may be worried somebody is going to say something negative. However, it is better to address the issue than to continue doing something that is, for example, upsetting your patient. Giving feedback is also an important skill, as you need to be aware of how your state of mind and personal attitudes might be influencing the feedback. It can be tempting to be very positive to avoid conflict; however, this will not be helpful if it is not honest. However, if you are too negative, you run the chance of the person totally disengaging with you and of knocking their self-esteem. It is usually helpful to start and end on a positive note when giving feedback in order to give people a sense of empowerment – it is all about balancing the negatives with the positives.

Activity 6.5	*Communication*

Ask one of your student nurse colleagues to give you a detailed account of their last night out on the town. Once they have finished, try to summarise it back to them using your own words. Consider with your colleague how successful you were at gathering the information and summarising.

- Do you think you listened more attentively?
- If so, what was different?

You can practise this technique in handovers when on clinical learning experience.

There is no outline answer for this activity.

Through genuinely hearing a patient who is mentally distressed you are more able to work with them as a unique individual and empower them in collaborating in the planning of their own care. Poor listening skills can result in a patient being confused and anxious, and can even lead to mistakes happening. Using listening skills, questioning skills and the observation of cues will aid you in building the therapeutic relationship.

We all have the potential to create barriers to effective listening; it often happens unconsciously even when we are trying our best to 'help'; our need to help the person in itself can manifest in a way that creates a barrier. The need people have to help or seem helpful might lead to an unaware preoccupation with what their next question will be or increased self-consciousness (McCabe and Timmins, 2006). Becoming overwhelmed with self-consciousness can deflect from the focus on the other person (Underman Boggs, 2007a). Having mentioned a lot about being self-aware in this chapter, the previous sentence may seem a little at odds with this. Being aware that you can become self-conscious and working on that within yourself can be helpful for situations that you find difficult.

The power of touch

The issue of physical touching is often a tricky one, particularly in mental health when it is not uncommon to be working with service users who have suffered physical abuse. There is no denying the power of touch in communicating with people. Touch can demonstrate empathy and offer much comfort and security (Bowers et al., 2009). Touch can even replace the spoken word when one is unable to find the right words to convey the levels of sympathy that a given situation deserves (Chambers and Ryder, 2009). Yet the incredible power of touch can be equally as powerful when misinterpreted, and it could lead you into a lot of trouble if you do not use it appropriately – the use of skills in self-awareness here is critical. The experience of touch for individuals varies so greatly that it is difficult to suggest any general rules; however, if somebody is agitated or angry, then it is a bad idea to invade their personal space by touching them, and you run the risk of a punch on the nose.

Questioning skills

Questioning is another key communication skill that you must develop in order to facilitate a successful therapeutic relationship with patients. Questioning is the main way of getting the information we need from patients in order to collaborate on their care planning. It is important to strike a balance between asking enough questions so that the patient is feeling listened to but not so many that at an intervention begins to feel like an interrogation.

In order to effectively gather information from patients you need to utilise three different question types: open, closed and circular questions.

Open questions

Open questions are very important, particularly in the initial stages of an interaction. An example of a good initial open question could be (after initial introductions): 'Can you tell me what has brought you here today?' An open question will very often start with a 'can you tell me about' or 'how', 'what', 'where', 'when', 'in what way'. You can see how these questions are not at all specific, giving the patient the opportunity to respond in a variety of different ways. Open questions give the patient the opportunity to tell their story and can provide a lot of information that can easily be missed if you launch straight into very closed 'yes' or 'no' questions (Dickson and Hargie, 2006). An open question provides the patient with the opportunity to talk about their own individual experience of the issue rather than you making your own subjective interpretation. This can reduce your influence on the direction of the patient's response and can also demonstrate that you have time to listen, which can help you to build rapport.

Open questions can provide broad information that you may need. Next you may need to clarify points and elicit some specific information based on some of the content in the broad response from the patient. Now you can use slightly more focused open-ended questions. For example, when responding to your open questions a patient may mention that they have had a lot of difficulty sleeping. You might then ask a focused question such as: 'You mentioned that you are having some difficulty with sleeping. Can you tell me a bit more about this?'

Closed questions

Closed questions are used to get a very specific response. For example, to gain a crucial piece of information once a patient has talked openly about their feelings prior to a suicide attempt, you might ask whether they intended to end their life. Or to a patient who is depressed, malnourished and who has said they lack any appetite, you might ask 'When did you last eat?', 'Did you manage to finish your meal?' or 'Have you ever felt like this before?'

Closed questioning can be extremely useful in certain mental health interactions, for example with very depressed or psychotic patients, who are struggling to concentrate on what is being said because they are preoccupied with their own thoughts. Such patients may find it easier to respond to simple 'yes' or 'no' questions. At the other extreme, closed questioning may be helpful with a manic patient who is over-stimulated and talking so much that it is difficult for you to ask open questions because they are jumping to a different idea before answering your question.

Crisis or emergency situations will often warrant the use of closed questioning because you might need answers to very specific questions in order to provide immediate help or treatment. Always try to remember that the type of question you use should be related to the current ability of the patient to answer.

It is important to remember when working on a busy ward that it is very easy for nurses to slip into closed questioning habits in order to take control of interactions and get answers quickly. This can come across to the patient as a one-sided checklisting operation and goes against everything discussed regarding active listening to engage the patient. When working within a mental health setting you can easily miss out on vital information, which can result in poorer care provision. This would not be a person-centred approach to communication; it could instead be seen as a task-centred approach (Bowers et al., 2009).

Circular questioning

Circular questioning techniques can help you understand the interpersonal impact of an individual's illness. Rather than exploring the illness itself it is about exploring the impact the illness has on each member of the patient's family and/or carers. This can help you to identify patterns of behaviour – both functional and dysfunctional – between family members, in order to aid in helping the family discover ways of improving their interactions and better supporting each other. This fairly advanced technique is often carried out by highly qualified systemic family therapists and perhaps is beyond the realms of this chapter to explain in detail – there are plenty of web resources if you want to follow this up. As identified already, the therapeutic alliance is about working with the whole person including family members, and so the use of circular questioning to understand what is happening between people in the system can help in a trained person's work with patients.

Activity 6.6   **Critical thinking**

Try to identify the following active listening questions as open, open-focused or closed:

- Would you like to have something to eat now or later on?
- How are you?
- You mentioned that you are worried that somebody has been spying on you. Could you tell me why you think that might be happening?
- How have you been feeling since starting the new medication?
- Has our meeting today been useful to you?
- Are you upset?
- Is there anything that you think your mum could have done differently last night?
- What has helped when you have felt like this in the past?
- Did you intend to end your life?
- What were your feelings just prior to taking the overdose?
- What would you like to talk about today?
- How did you get on with the plan that we developed together last week?

continued overleaf . . .

---

continued . . .

- You mentioned that you have been having some trouble with your sleep; can you tell me some more about this?
- What are your thoughts about having a short admission to hospital?
- As a brother, what is your perspective on how things have been at home?

There is an outline answer at the end of the chapter.

Considered use of open and closed questions appears to be the most appropriate option for patient-centred therapeutic relationships. After allowing a patient time and space to respond to an open question, you might begin to ask more focused clarifying or closed questions. This technique is called **funnelling** and allows us get specific information we need while encouraging patients to tell their story and share their interpretation of what they are experiencing (Goldberg and Murray, 2006). This demonstrates to patients that you are genuinely interested in them and should result in the patient feeling valued and cared for as a unique individual. Like any other aspect of communication it is important to consider your approach before you speak to the patient; however, you also need to adapt your style in accordance with how the interaction develops.

Paralinguistics

Paralinguistics are the non-verbal communication components – such as tone, pitch, volume, accent and speed of the voice – that appear alongside verbal communication (McCabe and Timmins, 2006). Have you ever found yourself saying 'It's not what you said but how you said it'? Paralinguistics can be used to demonstrate our emotions. This means that they can greatly alter the meaning of the spoken word, even contradicting the content of what is said through, for example, the use of a sarcastic tone.

Activity 6.7   *Critical thinking*

Try watching 10 or 15 minutes of a film on your own or with any number of people. It is very important that you have not seen the film before and that you have the volume turned right down so that all you can do is observe the non-verbal behaviour.

- Write down all the emotions you see and the responses to those emotions. If you undertake this activity with a colleague, you can compare your interpretations before watching the film back with the volume reinstated so that you can hear what is going on.
- Make a note of your accuracy of picking up on the non-verbal communication and see how that matches with other people's interpretations.

There is no outline answer provided for this activity.

Through carrying out Activity 6.7 you may have realised how paralinguistics can have a massive impact on how even a simple statement or message is interpreted. It can help you to be aware of paralinguistics not only in your own communication but in that of your patients (Gordon et al., 2006). You might meet a patient who is saying all the right things, but something in the way in which they convey the information to you suggests that under the surface there is more going on for the person than they are willing to share with you verbally.

Have you ever had a row with somebody? Most of us have. What is normally the first thing to change in the interaction as it starts to become angry? Is it the words used? Or is it how you say the words? In an argument the volume begins to rise alongside the pitch of your voice long before you get to the point of telling the other person to go away or personally insulting them.

Accents can also cause issues when communicating. For example, a person who comes from a culture or place with a very strong accent and with a high volume and pitched tone could be perceived by somebody from a different culture or geographical place as being rude or pushy. Many unpleasant rows or misinterpretations in communicating might be avoided if people could develop an awareness of paralinguistics and use them to their advantage rather than dis-advantage when interacting.

Empathy

Empathy is a core element to a successful therapeutic relationship because it provides the patient with the feeling that they have been heard and that you genuinely understand their experience from their individual perspective.

Baron-Cohen (2003) describes empathy as the ability to:

> *spontaneously and naturally tune into another person's thoughts and feelings, whatever these might be. There are two major elements to empathy. The first is the cognitive component: Understanding the other's feelings and the ability to take their perspective. The second element to empathy is the affective component. This is an observer's appropriate emotional response to another person's emotional state.*

Empathy can give nurses the ability to maintain a sense of self by objectively acknowledging and perceiving a patient's distress without owning it. Owning a patient's difficulties can lead to a nurse feeling completely overwhelmed and losing a sense of their own identity in the relationship. This is often called over-involvement (Newman, 2007). Remember that a patient's feelings belong to them and not to you. You can demonstrate empathy in many verbal and non-verbal ways. Active listening demonstrates empathy, and it can be very useful to drop into your interactions verbal empathic responses such as 'What you are describing sounds as though it must have been a terrible experience for you'. By doing this you are validating the issue for the patient, and this can generate a sense of genuineness in the relationship within the patient (Moss, 2008).

Basic empathy can be described as patient-centred communication. It is essential for helping relationships and establishing rapport and trust. It is particularly appropriate when working with people who are mentally distressed because relationships in these settings are very often emo-tionally intense (Bowers et al., 2009). As nurses working with mental distress, you might often need to try to reduce anxiety, de-escalate anger, and engage people who may have been stigmatised, abused and poorly treated by health professionals in the past. You can achieve a good level of basic empathy through your use of active listening skills, including empathic responses and questioning.

Professional boundaries and self-disclosure

Boundaries can be seen as interpersonal limits on what is acceptable within the confines of the therapeutic relationship. Professional boundaries are vital for establishing and maintaining the relationship effectively. Having an awareness and understanding of these boundaries will protect and benefit both you as the nurse and the patient (Churchill, 2011). For professional boundaries to be successful you need to be consistent in maintaining them. The patient may not always be aware of the boundaries due to vulnerability and other emotional needs. Boundaries can include the time, place, purpose, length of contact time and rights to confidentiality. They can also include who might be involved in provision of care for the patient and can be agreed upon very early on in the relationship (Clarkson, 2003). Boundaries can also protect the vulnerable patient from becoming harmed through misinterpretation of what they might expect from the relationship (Underman Boggs, 2007c). For example, imagine if you were to regularly stay longer with the patient than originally agreed and began to spend a lot of time talking about things you did at the weekend. The focus can move away from a therapeutic relationship to something perceived by the lonely patient as a friendship. How do you think the patient will feel when, for example, you change jobs? As a nurse you need to continually reflect upon the relationships that you build with your patients, and if you think the boundaries are becoming blurred, speak to a supervisor or senior colleague for support. It is worth mentioning here a little more about self-disclosure – it is not uncommon for patients to ask personal questions about you, such as 'Do you have any children?', 'Are you married?', 'How long have you been a nurse?' Giving a brief answer to such questions and then returning to the focus of the interaction is generally fine. If there is something inside you telling you that you are not comfortable sharing some information about yourself, then it is your right not to. You can redirect by saying something along the lines of 'I would prefer to use the time we have to talk about you.' Sometimes use of appropriate self-disclosure can help you in developing the relationship that is personalised and human (Kagan and Evans, 1995). You are better able to demonstrate your professional conduct as a nurse through your awareness of boundaries.

Case study

A patient called Jimmy arrives at an A&E department having self-injured (he has made some superficial lacerations to his left wrist). Julie, the new staff nurse, feels a bit uncomfortable about dealing with him because she has never met somebody who has done anything like that before. She also feels that somebody else who has fallen off their bike and hurt their leg should have preference. Through reflecting on her thoughts Julie realises her thoughts about self-injury are perhaps clouding her judgement, and so she decides to put her own thoughts to one side and treat Jimmy as she would anyone else. When she starts talking to him she begins to feel very sorry for him due to his recent difficulties – in fact, his story very much reminds her of a friend. As the intervention appears to be going very well, Julie begins to feel pleased with herself and how she has coped. Jimmy tells Julie how good she has been and begins asking her about how she got in to nursing. Julie happily

continued opposite . . .

continued . . .

answers him. She feels relieved to talk about herself as it is a bit easier than talking about Jimmy's complex issues. It is also quite nice for a patient to take an interest for a change. Jimmy asks a few other questions about where Julie grew up, and it turns out he knows a few of the people she went to school with. Julie begins to talk about a few of these people and what they are doing with themselves now. She also mentions how another friend of hers has struggled like Jimmy and how there should be much more help available for people in his position. Jimmy becomes upset and says he has never met anybody so kind. Julie feels flattered that Jimmy finds her a good nurse and says that he can come back and see her if ever he is struggling in the future.

Activity 6.8	Critical thinking

In the case study:

- What do you believe Julie did well?
- Where do you think Julie may have got into difficulty?
- How might Julie have handled this situation differently?

An outline answer is given at the end of the chapter.

Barriers to effective communication and relating

We have discussed how verbal and non-verbal communication skills are fundamental to the role of a nurse, how they enable nurses to develop rapport and are the foundations of a therapeutic relationship. We have also discussed how lacking these skills can lead to barriers in a nurse's work with patients. We have given some thought to barriers that can exist within the nurse and within the patient. We might also here consider barriers that can exist within the environment.

The development of a therapeutic alliance between nurse, patient and carers is essential and often at odds with service design. With an ever-increasing population and various government targets to hit, it can often feel as though the emphasis is on quantity rather than quality. This can all have an impact on the therapeutic relationship, and patient care can simply become automated – very task orientated. This poses the risk of being at odds with the patient-centred approach of treating patients as unique individuals (Martin, 1998).

The Mental Health Act and its impact

When working with those who are mentally distressed you may come across people who are subject to a section of the Mental Health Act, meaning that they may be detained in hospital against their will. This evokes a massive barrier that can deeply affect the dynamic of the relationship and can feel dramatically at odds with humanistic psychological theories. You may meet a patient who has been sectioned in the past, and the unconscious dynamics of the relationship would certainly need to be considered here. On a busy acute inpatient setting with somebody who is under section and detained against their will, it may feel to them, and even to you, as if there is a very unequal balance of power. It is not only with patients detained under the Mental Health Act that the unequal power relationship between nurse and patient rests. Sociological factors and influences can affect relationships with patients. An example of this is the socially constructed idea that when we go into hospital we go to receive care as a patient. This has the potential to place an individual in the role of dependency and disempowering them (Underman Boggs, 2007a).

If you consider some of the psychological principles discussed earlier in this chapter and apply those to each interaction, you might be better equipped to maximise on a patient's strengths as an individual. This can help prevent poor engagement in the therapeutic relationship due to the patient's perception that they are dependent on you and the service. The aim is to promote autonomy through working in partnership with patients and their carers rather than seeing them as passive recipients of care (Simpson and Brennan, 2009).

Communicating in difficult situations

We have probably all been involved in an interaction with a person or a group of people where we have felt incredibly uncomfortable and wonder what on earth we are going to do to resolve the issue. Situations when a person is very angry immediately spring to mind; however, what each individual finds difficult can vary greatly because of past experiences and levels of self-confidence. Difficult situations are often perceived as difficult because of the high expression of emotion, a perceived lack of communication ability and cultural differences (Gamble, 2006). Throughout this chapter we have discussed self-awareness and how some understanding of psychological principles from the likes of Sigmund Freud and Carl Rogers can help nurses manage interactions that they feel uncomfortable with. That is all very well, but when you are put on the spot in a real situation you are not always prepared, and textbook theories will feel a million miles away. Imagine for a moment an angry relative who is demanding answers on why their brother has had to wait so long to be seen. Through learning to manage intense feelings of anxiety in yourself you are able to cope better with somebody else who is in a state of emotional distress and unable to communicate in an effective manner (Gamble, 2006).

When you find a situation difficult it can lead to you becoming avoidant or communicating ineffectively. As well as being unhelpful to the patient it can affect your own level of professional confidence, as you feel you are unable to manage where others can. Managing our own anxieties means you can move away from wanting the situation to end because of how it is making you feel to focus more on the experience of the patient (McCabe and Timmins, 2006).

A really useful way of working on your communication skills in difficult situations is the use of role play as both a nurse and a patient. Try playing out the scenario of a situation that you would find difficult. Through playing the role of the patient who is trying to communicate with a nurse, you may be able to identify with the patient's feelings. Think of a nurse who has really impressed you because of their ability to demonstrate confidence, listening skills, empathy and professionalism and observe them in practice. You could also think of a nurse whom you are not quite so impressed with and consider how they might create barriers to effective communication.

Resolving conflict

Difficult situations will often arise with perceived conflicts with a nurse, patient or carer and are a natural part of human relationships. For example, you might enter into an interaction with an idea about what the conflict is about, and the other person might have a different idea about the conflict. This highlights the importance of gaining an understanding of both your own and the other person's view of the issues in order to begin resolving the conflict. Conflict needs to be dealt with very clearly in terms of how you communicate and can be viewed as a warning that something needs to be addressed within the therapeutic alliance. If you do not assertively deal with a conflict, the therapeutic relationship may become stuck and the relationship will move away from helping an individual with their issues and focus more on the conflict (McCabe, 2002). To effectively manage conflict as nurses you need to develop your skills in assertiveness. Assertiveness in nursing practice can be demonstrated through setting goals, acting on those goals in a clear and consistent manner, and taking responsibility for the consequences of actions. Assertiveness is also about standing up for the right of others as well as our own rights. Underman Boggs (2007c) identify four different personal responses to conflict. Have a look at each one and take a moment to reflect upon the response that you are most likely to take to conflict.

Avoidance

People often avoid conflict because it makes them feel very uncomfortable, but avoidance can lead to a conflict not being resolved and an escalation of the issues. Avoidance can also be used positively in situations where addressing the conflict is a higher risk than resolving it. An example of positive avoidance might be avoiding your boss who happens to be in a bad mood and is going to yell at you because you forgot to buy some milk on your way into work. You might know very well that your boss is just in a bad mood anyway and that normally he would not care about the milk issue. To get into a row with him while he is in a bad mood is not worth the energy on your part. However, when he is calmer you might have a chat with him about his mood swings.

Accommodation

This is the situation when you want to quickly sort out the conflict. This response is not very assertive because it is often characterised by giving in to something to gain a quiet life. This approach will not usually deal with the issue. It can be useful when the issue means a lot to the other person but makes little difference to you or anyone else either way.

Competition

This response to conflict is very often characterised by a power struggle when the respondent is unwilling to compromise and can appear quite aggressive. This response can come across as authoritative and will often escalate conflict and/or cause great stress to the other party. It is not a very positive way to manage conflict.

Collaboration

This is a solution-focused response to conflict whereby both people involved attempt to work towards a solution systematically. Those involved identify the issue and confront it, acknowledge each other's thoughts and feelings while trying to solve the problem. This is the best approach to managing conflict.

Now consider some principles for effective conflict resolution that aim to respect the individual and demonstrate genuineness from you as a nurse. These may be applied to any conflictive situation.

Identify the issue that is causing conflict

Identify the issue that is causing the conflict as early as possible.

Self-awareness

Be aware of how you typically respond to conflict and so be able to recognise when a patient or carer is behaving in a way that invokes a response that is poor in terms of effective communication – you can then have more control. Through self-awareness you are more likely to be able to validate the person's feelings. Making use of empathetic statements is one example of how to do this. If a patient is disappointed or angry, allowing space for the patient to express their anger or disappointment without taking it personally can help. Remember to be assertive; if you avoid conflict by making a promise you cannot deliver, it is highly likely that it will come back to bite you or a poor unsuspecting colleague.

Remain focused on the issue

Concentrate on the identified issue and do not bring up past problems that may have occurred in your relationship, as these can escalate the emotions and hinder you in identifying and solving the conflict in question. Try to appreciate why the other person took the position they did.

Identify possible options

Do not try to solve the issue immediately – look at the range of options available and work collaboratively through the options until you can both agree on something that might be a work-able solution. Stay calm and focused on the desire to resolve the patient's problem.

Scenario

You are about to see the mother of 29-year-old David, who was admitted to a mental health ward a few weeks ago. He has a diagnosis of schizophrenia and agreed to start taking the anti-psychotic medication that he had stopped prior to becoming unwell. He has also agreed to engage in psychological therapy sessions that are held at the hospital. Prior to his admission to hospital, David had been staying with his alcohol-dependent brother Adam. Adam had agreed to care for him, but was spending all his money on drink and keeping David quiet with alcohol. David was underweight, and his liver function tests were deranged on admission, suggesting he had been drinking quite heavily. David's mental distress has improved; however, he is still experiencing hallucinations and becomes distressed by his 'visions' very frequently, both day and night. He requires support with all daily activities including eating, drinking, washing and changing clothes because of confusion and

continued opposite . . .

continued . . .

disorientation. David's mother wants him discharged to her care at her house 40 miles away; the multidisciplinary team are very worried about this idea and believe that at present David will need continuing nursing care. The mother has a full-time job in a café; her husband – David's father – is at home, unemployed and a heavy drinker. David says that he does not mind either way. David's mother has become very angry in the past when she has wanted to take David home and the team has not felt he is ready.

Activity 6.9 *Decision making*

- In the case study, what conflicts can you identify?
- What are the issues? Should David go and stay with his mother?
- How might we approach managing a conflict like this?
- What communication skills might be useful in speaking to David's mother?

An outline answer is given at the end of the chapter.

Through being assertive you are better able to manage a situation such as the one in the scenario above. You can use many of the communication skills listed in this chapter to aid you in working with anger, such as identifying non-verbal cues of anger and by naming it, saying something like 'You appear tense and angry' and then allowing the person some space to express why they might feel angry, followed up by an empathic statement such as 'I can see how this would make you feel very angry'. This acknowledges that the individual is angry and that you can see why they are angry, at which point you might be ready to start exploring the causes and possible options for resolving the issue causing them such anger. Remember not to use leading questions when exploring the anger; try to stick to open questioning to allow the patient to explore their own feelings, and then summarise what they have told you.

It is important to remember that conflict is not always a negative thing and that it can be your feelings about conflict rather than conflict itself that you want to avoid. Have you ever dealt with something that has been worrying you for some time and found that once you have dealt with it you feel much better? It is highly likely that the situation you dealt with was difficult for you to face because it involved something that you perceived as a conflict, when in reality the thought (anxiety) of dealing with it was worse than the reality. When a conflict has been resolved, a relationship can feel much healthier and ready to move on to a subsequent stage.

Chapter summary

In this chapter we have established that evolving as an expert communicator is absolutely fundamental to our role as a nurse in order to develop, maintain and end relationships with people who are experiencing mental distress.

continued overleaf . . .

continued . . . •

We have discussed how, in order to do this, we can use reflection and principles from psychological theories to develop very high levels of self-awareness in order to better understand ourselves and how we respond when interacting with others.

This can equip us with the ability to better utilise practical skills such as active listening, questioning and the therapeutic use of ourselves to help people in a way that respects them as unique and whole individuals.

By being mindful of the ideas discussed in this chapter, both in work and in the wider context of our lives, we can develop skills that can not only benefit others but also reduce our own levels of stress.

Activities: brief outline answers

Activity 6.3: Critical thinking (page 102)

The nurse is feeling responsible for making the patient happy and has perhaps become over-involved with her. The nurse should discuss this case and her feelings with her clinical supervisor at the earliest opportunity.

Activity 6.4: Communication (page 105)

The 90-degree angle will normally feel less threatening. Sitting side by side will often feel very impersonal and non-connected.

Activity 6.6: Critical thinking (pages 109–10)

Question	Question type
Would you like to have something to eat now or later on?	Open-focused
How are you?	Open
You mentioned that you are worried that somebody has been spying on you. Could you tell me why you think that might be happening?	Open-focused
How have you been feeling since starting the new medication?	Open-focused
Has our meeting today been useful to you?	Closed
Are you upset?	Closed
Is there anything that you think your mum could have done differently last night?	Open-focused
What has helped when you have felt like this in the past?	Open-focused

Question	Question type
Did you intend to end your life?	Closed
What were your feelings just prior to taking the overdose?	Open-focused
What would you like to talk about today?	Open
How did you get on with the plan that we developed together last week?	Open-focused
You mentioned that you have been having some trouble with your sleep; can you tell me some more about this?	Open-focused
What are your thoughts about having a short admission to hospital?	Open-focused
As a brother, what is your perspective on how things have been at home?	Open

Activity 6.8: Critical thinking (page 113)

Julie does well by initially putting to one side her own beliefs about who should get preference for treatment by being reflective. She gets into difficulty when she is complimented on her skills as a nurse, and her need to feel good clouds her judgment in communicating with the patient. This leads to her disclosing lots of information about herself and perhaps stepping over her professional boundaries as a nurse. Julie may want to reflect upon this scenario with her supervisor and consider how, although it is nice to be complimented, she must try to maintain some objectivity when working with people in order to protect both herself and the patient.

Activity 6.9: Decision making (page 117)

David is at high risk of neglect if he stays with his brother, so this is not really an option. David's mum may be unable to care for him at home adequately due to her illness and the fact that she works full-time; however, this is what she wants. Alcohol has been an issue, and David's father is at home drinking heavily. The nursing team feel reluctant to discharge him. David's wishes seem to have been ignored. The best way forward might be for David to stay in hospital. A very clear and honest rationale for his continued stay would need to be reached and explained to all. Valuing the role of David's mother by including her in the decision-making process as much as possible will go some way to reducing her anger at the situation.

Further reading

Arnold, E and Underman Boggs, K (2011) *Interpersonal relationships: professional communication skills for nurses*, 6th edn. St Louis, MO: Saunders Elsevier.

This is a cracking book if you want a more in-depth look at the themes discussed within this chapter.

Bach, S and Grant, A (2009) *Communication and interpersonal skills for nurses*, Exeter: Learning Matters.

A clear and concise guide with good learning activities.

Useful websites

www.gp-training.net/training/communication_skills/calgary/guide.htm

This is a useful guide regarding the communication process.

www.thecounsellorsguide.co.uk/

This site has lots of information that builds on the themes discussed within this chapter.

http://changingminds.org/index.htm

This is another website full of useful information and links.

Chapter 7
Assessing mental health needs

Steven Trenoweth

continued . . .

7. All nurses must be able to recognise and interpret signs of normal and deteriorating mental and physical health and respond promptly to maintain or improve the health and comfort of the service user, acting to keep them and others safe.

Domain 4: Leadership, management and team working

4. All nurses must be self-aware and recognise how their own values, principles and assumptions may affect their practice. They must maintain their own personal and professional development, learning from experience, through supervision, feedback, reflection and evaluation.

NMC Essential Skills Clusters

This chapter will address the following ESCs:

Cluster: Organisational aspects of care

9. People can trust the newly registered graduate nurse to treat them as partners and work with them to make a holistic and systematic assessment of their needs; to develop a personalised plan that is based on mutual understanding and respect for their individual situation promoting health and well-being, minimising risk of harm and promoting their safety at all times.

By the second progression point:

9. Undertakes the assessment of physical, emotional, psychological, social, cultural and spiritual needs, including risk factors by working with the person and records, shares and responds to clear indicators and signs.

By entry to the register:

12. In partnership with the person, their carers and their families, makes a holistic, person centred and systematic assessment of physical, emotional, psychological, social, cultural and spiritual needs, including risk, and together develops a comprehensive personalised plan of nursing care.

Chapter aims

By the end of this chapter, you should be able to:

- understand the methods and principles of assessing mental health needs;
- distinguish between objective, subjective and functional assessments;
- understand and describe the criteria for comprehensive and holistic assessments of the person experiencing mental ill health;
- discuss the importance of a strengths-oriented assessment.

Introduction

In this chapter we explore the different methods of attempting to understand the problems and needs of an individual who may be experiencing mental ill health. In making an assessment we need to think about all aspects of the person's health and social functioning, and at the same time make sure we listen to the person and seek their views on their current difficulties. This is because, as we saw in Chapter 1, the needs of a person experiencing mental ill health can be complex, encompassing all holistic dimensions of self.

We first look at the different methods of assessing mental health needs, before moving on to identify the principles of good practice in assessment. We then examine comprehensive and holistic assessments, including an examination of mental state. As assessments tend to focus on deficits, it is also vital to consider the abilities that a person has by undertaking 'strengths' oriented assessments. In this way, we can begin to understand the needs of someone experiencing mental health problems in order that we may be able to more fully respond to their particular needs and situation.

Methods of assessment

In Chapter 6, we discussed the importance of communicating and relating to people with mental health problems. Such skills are vital throughout the assessment process. Assessments must be service-user centred, and appropriate communication skills should be used to encourage the individual to 'tell their personal story' (Launer, 2002).

Activity 7.1   *Communication*

Think about how you might go about asking a person experiencing mental ill health or in mental distress to tell their personal story. What questions might you ask? How might you pose questions? How would you conduct yourself? That is, how would you communicate? You may want to refresh your memory by looking back at Chapter 6.

An outline answer is given at the end of the chapter.

Self-assessment, based on what a person says about themselves and their abilities, is important in the assessment process. It allows the individual to identify the issues that they see as problematic and that they are concerned about. There are many techniques that can be used to facilitate self-assessment, such as encouraging the person to keep a journal or diary relating to their thoughts, feelings and behaviours, and self-rating assessment tools. What is crucial, however, is that the nurse ensures that the person is able and willing to collect such data and that it is comprehensible and not a difficult or time-consuming task for the person.

Obviously, the assessment process will involve the use of questions, which can vary according to the degree of structure that they impose. Sometimes it will involve the use of open questions (broad questions that allow the respondent to answer in a manner of their own choosing) and closed questions (questions that invite a short answer, e.g. yes or no). Sometimes assessments can be very informal (such as those structured around a conversation) or quite formal (such as those structured around a particular assessment tool). Clinical guidelines issued by NICE relating to mental distress recognise, quite accurately, that most people with mental health or psychological problems are cared for in primary care settings. As such, there is a need for all nurses who work in primary care, or on medical or surgical admission wards, to undertake a basic assessment of mental distress – referred to as *screening*. For example, in attempting to identify those who may be experiencing a depressive episode, NICE (2007) suggests the following brief screening questions to ascertain if treatment is warranted or if further specialist help needs to be sought.

- During the last month, have you been bothered by feeling down?
- During the last month, have you often been bothered by having little interest or pleasure in doing things?
- How well have you been sleeping lately?
- What's your appetite been like recently?

Activity 7.2   *Communication*

How are you?

Very often when making polite conversation we ask 'How are you?' This is a social convention, but it can be a very useful starting point for any health-care assessment. Technically, it is a global and open-ended question that the person is free to answer in any way they wish. So: 'How are you?'

An outline answer is given at the end of the chapter.

Now imagine for a moment that you feel you have many problems. Answering the question 'How are you?' is likely to be challenging for you. Where do you start? One of the challenges in mental health care is to assist the person experiencing mental distress to share their answer to this question in a way that is comprehensible to others so that we can help them rebuild their lives.

From a nursing point of view we must remember that whatever care we provide is focused on working with and alongside patients and service users. This is true with assessments, too. Nurses must provide clear information as to the purpose of the assessment. As far as possible, patients and service users must be seen as partners in this process. In the next section, we explore the reasons for this and why we must consider the underlying principles of the assessment process.

Principles of assessment

As we have seen from Chapter 3, there are many policies that currently influence the way in which mental health care is delivered. Central to this in contemporary mental health care, as we saw in Chapter 1, is the 'recovery model', which has found expression in the National Institute for Mental Health in England's *Recovery statement* (NIMHE, 2005b). 'Recovery' is seen not in terms of an absence of psychiatric symptoms, but in terms of helping people to live an empowered and personal meaningful life, as a valued member of a community.

Central to the notion of recovery is that of service user involvement, working in partnership and collaboration in all aspects of care (DH, 2006b), and this includes having an important voice in the assessment process, which should be collaborative, involving the person, their carer and family whenever appropriate and possible. This approach, stated in the Department of Health policy *The expert patient* (DH, 2001a), highlights notions of shared expertise and recognises that while health-care workers may have skills and knowledge in the delivery of evidence-based care, it is the individual service user who is ultimately the expert in what works for them.

In contemporary mental health care, however, there is often a focus on assessments that seek to identify the nature and extent of an individual's mental 'illness' via the establishment of a psychiatric diagnosis – the dominant paradigm in mainstream contemporary mental health care being the medical model. Psychiatry, as we mentioned in Chapter 1, is the branch of medicine that deals with the assessment and treatment of mental disorder. However, medical assessments that exclusively focus on symptom exploration for the purposes of psychiatric diagnosis may oversimplify the nature of an individual's distress and may not account for variations in individual experiences of mental distress; nor may they allow the individual to fully share their unique experiences. This may be disempowering to the individual, for their role may be seen in terms of providing the data that is used by another to form an opinion about their health status or illness. We must also remember that nurses in all fields must be able to provide care holistically, including health promotion and health education, rather than focusing on treating the medical symptoms of a disease (NMC 2010a).

Psychiatric diagnoses such as paranoid schizophrenia and bipolar affective disorder may mask perceptions of the individual as a whole person, particularly when an individual is defined in terms of their psychiatric 'status' – a 'schizophrenic', for example – and this is the essence of *labelling* (Goffman, 1963). When people are 'labelled' like this they are seen, and may come to see themselves, as being *ill* and requiring medical treatment to address the underlying pathology. It also encourages the view that the person experiencing mental distress is disabled because often such assessments tend to be focused on dysfunction and deficits rather than the strengths and abilities that the person may possess (this may also lead to perceptions that people experiencing mental distress are, and should be, passive recipients of care and treatment).

Look back at the case study about Sandra at the beginning of Chapter 1, on page 8, as it illustrates this point. It seems that the diabetic nurse specialist has made a number of assumptions based on the label that has been applied to Sandra. The nurse appears to assume that Sandra is not capable of remembering to take her medication because she is 'mentally ill'. This is clearly an assumption that people experiencing mental ill health are forgetful or feckless, or perhaps have a reckless attitude to their health and well-being. When one starts with such assumptions, one's assessments cannot be considered 'objective' and as such may be tainted by one's own biases and prejudices, which can affect the subsequent nursing care and treatment offered.

There is increasing recognition of the importance of attempting to understand the person's internal frame of reference (DH, 2006b) and also that the values that underpin professional mental health care must start with the service user's experience (Woodbridge and Fulford, 2004). This means seeking to capture personal narratives of mental distress, which involves:

> *gathering information and understandings about a client's inner and outer worlds from their frame of reference. It should be, as far as possible, a collaborative process in which the helper and the client try to identify what is going on and what is going wrong (and right too).*
> (Watkins 2001, p45)

Watkins here is also stating the importance of considering the strengths, talents, assets and abilities of an individual.

In attempting to understand a *client's inner and outer world* it is likely that we need to undertake wide-ranging assessments – those that are comprehensive and holistic and span the breadth of an individual's potential health and social care needs, and their abilities too (DH, 2006b). It is these kinds of assessment we will look at next. Crucially, however, the approach needs to be systematic and well organised in order to understand the various complexities of the issues facing the person in mental distress (Onega, 1991).

Comprehensive and holistic assessments

Activity 7.3 — *Reflection*

Spend a few moments thinking about what is meant by comprehensive and holistic assessments.

An outline answer is given at the end of the chapter.

Before we look in more detail at specific assessments in mental health care, it is important to clarify what is meant by objective, subjective and functional assessments – they are often referred to in general health care, but they have particular implications in mental health and psychiatric care.

'Objective' assessments are based on information that is collected in a neutral and unbiased way, and is often, but not exclusively, quantitative in nature. Importantly, such data is verifiable by another person. 'Objective' information can come from observations (such as vital signs, the individual's personal and medical history and physical examinations) or from an interview (such as the identification of symptoms that may lead to a psychiatric diagnosis). A blood pressure reading is an example of an objective assessment that is confirmable by another person.

'Subjective' data, however, refers to information that is of personal relevance to the individual, such as the person's views of their current difficulties and problems (Margereson et al., 2010). Information from subjective assessments is likely to be especially meaningful to the individual and should be recorded wherever possible in their own words to ensure the authenticity and representativeness of the service user's views.

'Functional' assessments refer to those assessments that aim to understand the person's ability and the deficits that may impair a person's ability to live their day-to-day life independently. Such deficits may be of a physical nature (such as a lack of mobility caused by arthritis) or result from cognitive or sensory impairment (such as a loss of short-term memory resulting from dementia) or related to environmental factors (such as a lack of easy access to public buildings for wheelchair users). Functional assessments are often undertaken by occupational therapists or psychologists and are an essential adjunct to nursing care.

Activity 7.4   *Critical thinking*

Which of the following are the results of objective, subjective or functional assessments?

- Blood pressure = 150/80.
- 'I feel I can't go on.'
- Pulse = 80 bpm.
- Sally needs to be reminded to wash her hands before preparing food.
- 'I'm much happier today.'
- Fred is partially sighted and needs written information in a large font size.

Answers are given at the end of the chapter.

It is very important that a wide range of comprehensive objective, subjective and functional health and social care assessments are undertaken in mental health care in order to obtain a full understanding of each individual (Phelan et al., 2001). Here it is important to avoid focusing too much on specific areas relating to what is thought be the individual's main 'problem', such as a psychiatric diagnosis. If one does, then a picture of the whole person may be lost, and one will not be able to see how various aspects of the person's health, life and functioning may be of relevance to a mental health problem the person may be experiencing.

Personal biography

When undertaking an assessment, an important starting point is the individual's *personal biography* in order to attempt to understand the current context of a person's life. It is important to capture essential contemporary biographical information, such as name, age, address, ethnicity/place of birth, current occupation and employment status, suitability and satisfaction with accommodation, financial issues (including receipt of benefits), marital status and next of kin, significant others, including children, and so forth. It will also be of interest to understand the ways in which the person asserts their individuality, such as through dietary preferences, hobbies and interests, and information about how the person expresses their cultural or religious identity.

Current stressors

It is vital to seek to establish details of the current stressors that the person feels they are currently facing. Stress often occurs as a result of the inability of an individual to respond and adjust to the environment or circumstances in which they find themselves (Butcher et al., 2008), and it is important to recognise the role that stress plays in the development and maintenance of mental distress, and its role in relapse. There may be many stressors that the person may be exposed to that can detrimentally affect an individual's mental health, and stress is a known risk variable for suicide (Barker, 2004). It is important to realise that people with mental health problems experience levels of social stress, such as stigma and discrimination, that may prolong their current troubles.

As we saw in Chapter 1, Zubin and Spring (1977) proposed the stress vulnerability model to account for the development of schizophrenia. Zubin and Spring (1977) argued that vulnerability to episodes of mental disorder is a function of neurobiological factors (such as genetic factors) and previous experiences, which can lead to a predisposition to mental ill health, but the risk of developing mental health problems is mediated by environmental and life stressors.

In 1967, Holmes and Rahe attempted to capture the impact that life events have on our health and well-being. Their 'Life Stress Inventory' gives an overview of some of the major life events, and is a method of capturing and quantifying the magnitude of change a person experiences in their life and the subsequent stress that may result. For example, 'death of a spouse' scores 100 on the scale, while minor problems with the law (e.g. getting a parking ticket) scores 11. Life events, such as having a baby or going on holiday, may be a time of great happiness but may also be accompanied by stress (these events score 39 and 13 respectively). Of course, life events may occur simultaneously and the resultant stress may be cumulative and compounded – the more life events stress, the greater the implications for our health. For example, a person who experiences the death of a spouse (scores 100) may also experience a major change in their financial state as a consequence (scores 38), a major change in their living conditions as they have to move home (scores 25). They might also experience a major change in their social activities (scores 18). The overall score for this person is therefore 181. A cumulative score of over 300 suggests a very high risk of developing a serious illness (80 per cent chance); between 150 and 299 suggests a 50 per cent chance of developing an illness; while those who score below 150 have only a slightly elevated risk.

Personal history

An important part of understanding the person is to review their *personal history*. This process attempts to understand the context of a person's life and their difficulties. This often establishes the backdrop to a person's current troubles and helps to reveal information relating to an individual's vulnerability (Zubin and Spring, 1977). Margereson et al. (2010) suggest that the assessment of personal history should include details of:

- previous episodes of mental ill health;
- previous history of risk (for example, violence, suicide attempts, drug use);
- previous medical/surgical history, including allergies and immunisation;

- previous treatment and nursing care, including prescribed medication (see below);
- relevant family history, including health conditions of parents, grandparents, siblings, children and grandchildren;
- social history, including social networks;
- previous intimate/personal relationships;
- history of education, vocational training and achievements;
- occupational history, including types of work and periods of employment.

It is vital, however, not to be too prescriptive and directive in obtaining such information, and steps should be taken to ask the person if there is anything they feel from their history that may have a bearing on their present experience of health and illness. In this sense, the assessment of personal history should be seen as the starting point of a subjective assessment (Margereson et al., 2010).

Current mental ill health

Mental distress is not an uncommon experience, and some of us may require treatment or referral to specialist services at some point in our lives, particularly if our distress becomes persistent or leads to functional impairment and undermines the quality of life or if we pose a risk to ourselves or to others.

Activity 7.5 *Critical thinking*

What issues do you think the nurse needs to take into consideration when making an assessment of a person's mental state?

An outline answer is given at the end of the chapter.

There are many factors that need to be taken into account when examining someone's mental state, and these centre around **mood**, appearance and behaviour, **cognition** and **perception**.

Mood

If you experience a mood disturbance, you may feel anxious or sad, or experience despair, anguish and guilt (feelings that often underlie depression). Alternatively, you may feel elated or euphoric (as in the case of manic episodes). It is possible, of course, for you to experience feelings of depression and mania alternately, such as in bipolar affective disorder (sometimes referred to as manic depression).

Some people may have persistent and disabling feelings of anxiety, worry, fear and panic. If someone has a specific fear of an environmental stimulus that is not currently harmful, then this is known as a phobia. Phobias are very common, and many people can lead their lives normally in spite of their fears. However, for people who have fears of open spaces or other people, their phobias can be extremely troublesome and can seriously undermine their quality of life. Anxiety may also result from persistent internal ruminations centring on problems the person feels they face. At such time, people may experience panic attacks, for example, particularly when they feel that they are helpless to do anything to solve a current crisis and that they have no control over the events that are the source of their distress.

Appearance and behaviour

An individual's appearance and behaviour can be a good indicator of the mental distress they may be experiencing. People who are low in mood, for example, may withdraw from social situations, and appear sad or tearful. It is not uncommon for them to demonstrate a slowness of movement or an increased reaction time when responding to questions. Alternatively, people who are elated may talk at a rapid rate, and at a higher volume, and appear excited or agitated and have an increased rate (pressure) and volume of speech, and be overactive, restless or agitated.

People who are experiencing anxiety may tremble or shake. They may be seen to pace around, finding it difficult to settle or rest. Sometimes an individual may exhibit repetitive behaviours that reduce levels of anxiety. For example, someone who has excessive worry over hygiene may demonstrate excessive hand washing, suggestive of an obsessive compulsive disorder. For some people who experience mental distress there may be a lack of motivation to attend to even the most basic of personal self-care or to their appearance or personal hygiene (Matthews and Trenoweth, 2008), which may not be in keeping with their usual routine.

Cognition

In assessing cognition one is interested in the way someone is thinking (the form of their thinking) and what they are thinking about (the content of their thoughts) (Barker, 2004). For example, a person's thought processes may be 'racing' as suggested by the speed at which they are talking. They may also jump between topics in a conversation, known as flight of ideas. Alternatively, a person may have trouble in understanding what is being said to them, and may be very slow in responding to questions, indicating impairment in the processing of information. They may also have difficulty in decision-making and problem solving, and this is particularly troublesome for people who have many life stressors requiring resolution. People who are said to be 'thought disordered' (a symptom that may be experienced in schizophrenia) may use words that are disconnected and form sentences in which the word order is jumbled up.

A person may lack an awareness of the significance or the extent of their mental ill health, and they may express ideas that appear strange to the listener. Such ideas may be completely impossible (known as delusions) or the person may believe that information in the public domain has personal significance for them (known as ideas of reference). Furthermore, some people may believe that they are being controlled by some external force or that particular people or groups of people, such as their neighbours, wish to harm them.

When someone is low in mood they may harbour negative beliefs about themselves or their situation. They may, for example, believe that they are worthless or that their future is bleak and hopeless. People may also have beliefs that they have a physical health problem, despite medical evidence to the contrary (this is known as hypochondriasis).

Perception

We have at least five senses – olfactory (smell), gustatory (taste), auditory (hearing), tactile (touch) and visual – and hallucinations can occur in any of them. It is important to recognise that hallucinations are very real sensations that a person experiences – they are not beliefs or illusions but experiences that occur in the absence of an external stimuli. It is also important to realise that hallucinations are not an uncommon human experience as a response to extreme or distressing circumstances. Visual hallucinations, for example, may occur in fevers or during times of extreme tiredness. Hallucinations become a mental health issue when a person regularly experiences such phenomena and particularly when this leads to distress (such as when a person 'hears' people making derogatory comments about them or gives a running commentary on their actions) or impedes their ability to live their lives.

Personal meaning

Think for a moment about what gives your life meaning. It is likely that you will think about something that helps you make sense of the world. For some people this may be a particular political ideology or religious belief. This may help you to make important connections with other people, such as a cultural group, and to express some common identity or solidarity with them. A life imbued with meaning has a sense of purpose and direction. There is a sense of forward momentum and achievement as one realises one's personal goals.

Often, people who experience a depressive episode feel that their life has no purpose or direction, that life is pointless and that the future is bleak. In short, they may feel that they are living a life that currently has no meaning – a known risk variable for suicide. An assessment of people experiencing mental distress needs to capture what gives the person's life meaning and whether the person feels that their life is currently imbued with a sense of purpose and direction. Do they feel that this has been lost recently? If so, how does the person account for this?

Understanding subjective experiences

In assessing mental distress, it is useful to undertake an initial wide-ranging (global) approach (Trenoweth and Allymamod, 2010), focusing on revealing the person's subjective experience of their current troubles. Fox and Gamble (2006) suggest that this can be facilitated by asking the following kinds of questions.

- *What* – e.g. What do you feel are the current problems for you?
- *When* – e.g. When does this affect you?
- *Where* – e.g. In what situations?
- *With* – e.g. Are there people who make the problems worse? Or better?
- *Why* – e.g. How do you account for your current problems?

In order to explore any significant issue in more detail, one might use 'funnelling' questions (Fox and Gamble, 2006).

- *Frequency* – e.g. How often does this occur?
- *Intensity* – e.g. On a scale of 0–10, where 10 is the most you can imagine and 0 is none at all, how problematic or troublesome is this for you?

- *Number* – e.g. How many times do you experience this? Do you notice any patterns?
- *Duration* – e.g. For how long do you experience this?

Psychiatric diagnosis

The diagnosis of psychiatric conditions is based on criteria established by a medical taxonomy, such as the *International classification of diseases* (*ICD-10*), published by the World Health Organization (WHO, 2004) or *Diagnostic and statistical manual* (*DSM-IV*), published by the American Psychiatric Association (APA, 2000). Such taxonomies cluster psychiatric symptoms into a hierarchically arranged diagnostic system with the aim of increasing the reliability of medical assessments (see Chapter 1).

The *ICD-10*, for example, classifies *mental and behavioural disorders* in the following way ('F' refers to the chapter of *ICD-10*, while the numeric code signifies particular disorders).

F00–F09   *Organic Mental Disorders (dementia, delirium, organic amnesia)*: disorders that are result of: Trauma to Brain; Degenerative Diseases of Nervous System; Toxic Substances.

F10–F19   *Psychoactive Substance Use (intoxication, harmful use, dependency, withdrawal)*: disorders that are the result of excessive and problematic use/misuse of alcohol and/or other substances that alter mental functioning and behaviour.

F20–F29   *Schizophrenia, Schizotypal and Delusional Disorders*: group of disorders characterised by marked impairment of 'reality', disturbances of thought and perception, and bizarre behaviour. Includes persistent delusional disorders and acute/transient psychotic disorders.

F30–F39   *Mood (Affective) Disorders*: includes depression, abnormal elation, or swings between the two (bipolar affective disorder).

F40–F48   *Neurotic, Stress-Related and Somatoform Disorders*: includes anxiety disorders, obsessive-compulsive disorders, and disorders that have physical symptoms believed to have a psychological cause.

F50–F59   *Behavioural Syndromes (eating disorder, sleeping disorders, sexual dysfunction)*: includes eating disorders and abuse of non-dependence producing substances (e.g. laxatives, painkillers).

F60–F69   *Disorders of Adult Personality*: deeply ingrained and long-standing pervasive patterns of maladaptive behaviours and cognitions that constitute immature and inappropriate ways of problem solving or coping. Contains a number of personality sub-groups (e.g. Emotionally Unstable Personality Disorder); habit and impulse disorders (such as pathological gambling, pathological fire-setting); and Gender Identity Disorders (e.g. transsexualism).

For example, paranoid schizophrenia is assigned the code F20.0. A diagnosis using the *ICD-10* will only be made by a psychiatrist if the person has satisfied the relevant criteria. In the case of paranoid schizophrenia, a person will have symptoms including persistent relatively stable, often paranoid delusions, usually accompanied by auditory hallucinations for a period of not less than one month.

Research summary: On being sane in insane places (Rosenhan's 1973 studies)

These famous psychological experiments were designed to see if psychiatrists could tell the difference between those who were 'sane' and those who were 'insane'. The first study involved eight people (from diverse backgrounds and with no current mental health problems) seeking to gain admission to different psychiatric hospitals in the USA.

The 'patients' complained that they had been hearing voices that were unfamiliar and often unclear but said 'empty', 'hollow', 'thud'. While false names were given, all other information that the person gave about their own lives was true. After being admitted, the 'patients' said that they no longer heard voices and participated in social activities, interacting as they would normally, making notes of their observations. Seven 'patients' were admitted with a diagnosis of 'schizophrenia', stayed for an average of 19 days, were given over 2,000 tablets and on discharge were seen to be 'in remission'. The normal behaviours of the 'patients' were often interpreted in terms of their diagnosis, with writing notes being seen as indicative of mental illness. Nursing records indicated that, for example, 'patient engages in writing behaviour'.

In the second study, the hospital staff, who were aware of the first study, were informed that more false 'patients' would be admitted to their ward over the coming months. They were asked to identify who they thought these were. About 10 per cent of admissions were judged by one psychiatrist and another staff member to be such 'false' patients. In fact, there were none.

Rosenhan felt that his studies demonstrated that psychiatrists could not reliably distinguish between those who were 'sane' and those who were 'insane'. He felt that the first study showed a failure by psychiatric staff to detect sanity, whereas the second showed a failure to detect insanity. He argued that it was the context of the hospital and the label of a psychiatric diagnosis that created the expectation that seemingly normal human behaviours were seen as pathological.

Medication

It is very important to elicit the person's understanding about any medication they may have been prescribed. Do they understand the rationale for the prescription? Do they feel the medication is helpful? Are they satisfied with the prescribed medication? Does the person understand the effects and side effects, and the need to take medication as prescribed?

Such understandings are likely to be related to an individual's concordance with prescribed treatment plans.

Activity 7.6   *Decision making*

Have you ever been prescribed medication by a GP but not taken it? Think of all the reasons why you might not take medication that has been prescribed for you.

An outline answer is given at the end of the chapter.

We may be dissatisfied with prescribed medication because we think it does not work. We may also feel that we lacked involvement in, and consent to, treatment decisions. For some people, this may lead to the use of unprescribed, over-the-counter or psychoactive substances (such as illicit drugs or alcohol) as a means to control symptoms. For example, there is evidence that elderly people may use/abuse alcohol as a means of controlling pain (Christensen et al., 2006). As such, it is important to understand if someone has been self-medicating and the possible reasons underlying their decision.

Suicide risk

Suicide is a complex issue. As suggested above, the experience of mental ill health and mental distress can, for some people, have implications for their personal safety. Where it is felt that a person may compromise their personal safety, then a comprehensive suicide risk assessment must be undertaken compassionately and sensitively (Watkins, 2001; Barker, 2004). It is important to recognise, for example, that most people who commit suicide have mental health problems (such as depression) at the time of their death and are under the influence of alcohol (Jenkins et al., 2008). However, social and environmental factors may also play a part, such as unemployment (ODPM, 2004). Suicide rates also increase with age and are higher among those who are single, widowed, divorced or separated (Watkins, 2001).

Research summary: Suicide risk factors

- Previous history of suicidal attempts.
- Family history of suicide.
- Negative view of the future – feelings of hopelessness, helplessness; does the person have any plans for the future?
- Mental health issues – especially depression, hallucinatory voices commanding self-harm or of persecution, alcohol/drug use.
- Social isolation – withdrawal, loss/lack of social support.
- Behaviour warning of suicidal intent – for example, procuring means of death, acts in anticipation of death, putting financial affairs in order, general behaviour at interview, plan to commit suicide.
- Current stressors – recent bereavement (especially of partner), relationship difficulties or other stressful events, financial problems, terminal illness, accommodation issues.

Source: Based on Barker, 2004; Cutcliffe and Barker, 2004

Any threats a service user makes regarding suicide (or any such concerns expressed by family members) must be actively followed up, and it is important to realise that suicidal intent is often communicated beforehand. Ideas of suicide may be explicit (and may include direct statements of wanting to die) or implicit (such as not seeing any possible future for themselves or discussing methods of suicide). A person who has a well-thought out, simple and highly lethal plan to end their life is at a significantly increased risk, and it is also important to carefully and sensitively explore with the suicidal person any such intentions they may have.

Functional assessments

As mentioned above, functional assessments seek to provide information with regard to a person's ability, motivation and potential to lead an independent life. Such assessments look at household or work-related skills and self-care ability, and identify specific deficits that impair performance. A risk assessment may be undertaken to ascertain if an individual's functional impairment may lead to injury or damage to their health.

The assessment of 'function' is a highly skilled activity usually carried out by occupational therapists. They examine a wide range of factors that may impair independence, social inclusion, access to work and leisure activities, education and mental health. The assessment may include a home visit by the occupational therapist. However, other specialist functional assessments are also carried out by other disciplines, such as physiotherapists, speech and language therapists and dieticians, who make an important contribution to identifying the individual's overall holistic health and social care needs.

The *DSM-IV TR* medical taxonomy includes an assessment of functioning – the Global Assessment of Functioning (GAF). This assessment (maximum score is 100 while the minimum score is 1) seeks to record the level of functioning for an individual who experiences mental distress. For example, people who are functioning extremely well across a range of activities score between 91 and 100; people who have moderate symptoms (such as occasional panic attacks) or have few friends, score between 51 and 60; and those whose behaviour is considerably influenced by delusions or hallucinations score 21 to 30.

Social assessments

Social situations can, for some people with mental health problems, be problematic. This might be due to: a loss of confidence or fears about how the person might be seen by others; concerns that other people might wish to do them harm; or, for people with long-standing and chronic problems, a loss of social skills.

It is important to remember that there are wide variations in people's interest and motivation to participate socially. Not everyone seeks out the company of others, for example. This is important, as any social assessment will need to appreciate an individual's desire for social contact and relationships, which may be unconnected with any mental distress they may be currently experiencing. Therefore, when conducting a social assessment, consideration must be given to any *changes* from the person's baseline behaviour, such as social withdrawal.

Physical health

As we saw in Chapter 4, there is much evidence that people with mental health problems have significantly poorer physical health than the general population. It is vital that an assessment of an individual's physical health is conducted to ensure that a person's mental distress is not connected to an underlying, and possibly undiagnosed, medical problem. The person's consent must always be obtained before any physical assessment, with a full explanation of what observations will be undertaken and the reasons for them, and any assessment must be carried out in an area that is quiet and offers privacy. Specific observations such as temperature, pulse respiration, blood pressure, height, weight, condition of skin, personal grooming and urinalysis should be undertaken and carefully recorded. Additional tests such as blood tests and electro-cardiograms may also be ordered, the latter being very important if a person is about to start anti-depressant medication, for example, as such drugs can have a **cardiotoxic** effect. The areas that should be covered when people with mental health problems have a physical check-up are outlined below.

- Calculation of body mass index, and/or body fat measurement and appropriate advice on healthy eating if the patient is obese.
- Comprehensive blood tests (e.g. serum electrolytes/complete blood counts (CBC)/liver function tests (LFT) and so forth).
- Cardiovascular assessment, including blood pressure check.
- Assessment of levels of exercise and advice, if appropriate.
- Cholesterol-level monitoring and advice on preventing cardiovascular disease, if appropriate.
- Urine analysis for sugar, with fasting blood sugar, if positive.
- Respiratory assessment, including peak flow readings.
- An assessment of smoking status, cessation advice, if appropriate.
- Annual influenza vaccination and other immunisations as appropriate.
- Regular preventive checks such as cervical smear, breast screening, testicular cancer and advice on self-monitoring.
- Advice of maintaining good sexual health and family planning with screening for associated infections, if appropriate.
- Assessment of alcohol use and other drug use with advice and brief intervention, if appropriate.

Assessing lifestyle issues

As we saw in Chapter 4, some, but by no means all, people who experience mental ill health also have lifestyle issues that affect their physical health. Sometimes this may be connected to their mental distress, and may even be a way of coping with their current problems. Here, we look at alcohol use, smoking, physical activity and diet.

Alcohol use

It is important to recognise the need for screening for the use and misuse of alcohol as the majority of people who use alcohol hazardously go undiagnosed (Trenoweth and Tobutt, 2009). Initial screening is likely to comprise essential biographical information relating to the person, along with information about levels and patterns of alcohol use (Scottish Executive, 2002). Such screening involves an assessment of the amount and pattern of a person's alcohol use. Current guidelines suggest that upper safe limits of alcohol are 14 units for women (with no more than 2–3 units a day) and 21 units of alcohol for men (with no more than 3–4 units a day). A unit is a half-pint of beer, a small glass of wine – 8 per cent **ABV**, 125ml, or 1 single shot of spirits – 25ml. A person should have two alcohol-free days a week. Anyone who drinks in excess of this is drinking in a potentially hazardous way and may be putting their health at risk. Some groups, such as pregnant women and those engaging in potentially dangerous activities (such as operating heavy machinery), should drink less or nothing at all.

If an individual's pattern of alcohol consumption is considered to be hazardous, then it may be appropriate to give feedback to the person about their levels of alcohol consumption; to offer advice about the benefits of sensible drinking; and to clarify the person's intentions to reduce their intake. If the person feels they would like support to reduce their alcohol use, then they may be referred for specialist treatment and support (HDA (Health Development Agency), 2002).

Smoking

Significantly more people with mental health problems smoke than in the general population, and this may account, at least in part, for an increased early mortality of this client group. Nurses need to be sensitive to people's freedom of choice to smoke, but also to be mindful of their role as promoters of health. It is important to establish a person's willingness, readiness and confidence in their ability to quit smoking. At the very least, an individual's use of cigarettes should be discussed with them, and smoking cessation advice should be provided when appropriate.

Feedback can be useful in supporting smoking cessation. Initially, the nurse may wish to work with the service user to identify patterns of their cigarette use and to establish how many cigarettes the person smokes and what may trigger the desire for a cigarette. It is important to consider when the first cigarette of the day is smoked and how long after waking. Those who tend to smoke immediately or soon after waking may be particularly physiologically dependent upon cigarettes.

Exercise and level of physical activity

An active lifestyle contributes to an overall positive sense of physical and mental health (NICE, 2007; Anstiss and Bromley 2010). For positive health benefits, adults should aim for at least 30 minutes of at least moderate intensity physical activity on five or more days of the week (DH, 2004b). A general assessment of activity levels is therefore important in a comprehensive and holistic assessment. However, the assessment of exercise and activity is a complex process and caution is advised. Nurses need to be mindful of risks associated with vigorous exercise, particularly among people who have not been active for a period of time. People who wish to take up exercise should be advised to consult appropriately trained staff, and to keep the intensity low at the start of any exercise programmes.

Weight, diet, fluid intake and nutrition

An assessment of nutritional intake and diet is vital in a comprehensive nursing assessment, and there is much that can be done to screen for potential problems before referral to specialist dietetic services. Everyone should eat a variety of at least five portions (at least 80 grams) of fruit and vegetables each day (DH, 2004c). Likewise, the nurse must ensure adequate fluid intake – between 1½ and 3 litres per day for an adult, which can include tea, coffee, juices and so forth in addition to water. However, it is important to be aware that some drinks can exacerbate a person's mental distress; for example, coffee or any highly caffeinated drinks should be avoided in a person who is experiencing stress or anxiety.

Such intake must be monitored carefully when a person is vulnerable to excessive calorific intake or malnutrition. The Body Mass Index (BMI) is a simple way of calculating a healthy weight for an individual's height (height in metres squared divided by weight in kilograms). There are many tools available on the Internet to calculate an individual's BMI score (for example, NHS Choices – see 'Useful websites' at the end of the chapter). Scores of less than 18.5 suggest that a person is likely to be underweight; scores between 18.5 and 24.9 suggest normal weight; while a score of between 25 and 30 suggests a person is overweight. Scores of 30.1 and over can indicate obesity. However, the BMI is not always a good guideline for healthy weight. It is not suitable for older people or children, and the muscle bulk of athletic people may artificially raise their BMI score. Other assessments can indicate if a person's weight suggests an increased health risk. A waist circumference of more than 80 cm for women and 94 cm for men is of concern, and those whose waist measures more than 88 cm for women and 102 cm for men have a significantly increased health risk.

It is important to remember that not everyone experiencing mental health problems may adopt an unhealthy lifestyle. Indeed, it is very important to remember that a comprehensive assessment also takes into consideration the strengths that a person has. As we shall see in the next section, strengths oriented assessments are vital to obtain a clear picture of a person's level of need and what they might be able to draw upon to help themselves to deal with their current troubles.

Strengths-oriented assessments

In undertaking an assessment of a person experiencing mental distress, it is very important to balance **problem-oriented assessments** with those that seek to capture skills and personal abilities, knowledge, talents, resilience and coping abilities, resources and opportunities. However, such assessments are infrequently undertaken in nursing practice, despite their obvious synergy with recovery models.

Much recent attention has been paid to the idea of Wellness and Recovery Action Planning (WRAP). It is based on the work of Mary Ellen Copeland and represents an important way in which nurses can enable and support the process of recovery (see 'Useful websites' at the end of this chapter). A key to this approach is to assist the person to keep track of their mental world, to be aware of their own needs and, crucially, to develop an action and crisis plan in the event of problems arising. Such a plan should capitalise on the strengths and abilities that a person can draw upon in improving their mental health during difficult times.

Case study

Fred is a 64-year-old man who has been diagnosed recently with ICD-10 F 34.1 Dysthymia. Fred's wife died two years ago and he says he can't seem to get over her death. They had been together for 40 years and were very close. They had no children, but Fred's wife was very fond of animals. When she died there were three dogs and six cats that shared their house. Following complaints from his neighbours, last year the RSPCA removed the animals from Fred's house as he was unable to look after them and they were malnourished and in poor physical health. Environmental Health Officers were also involved at this time to clean up Fred's house as it had been contaminated with animal faeces.

Since his wife died Fred says that he has been keeping himself to himself. He has no family locally and rarely leaves the house except to go to his GP's surgery to have his leg ulcer cared for. Fred has suffered for many years with angina but when asked about this he shrugs his shoulders, saying that it is something that he just has to live with.

The practice nurses have expressed their concern to the GP that Fred has apparently been neglecting his personal hygiene, increasing his use of alcohol, has an apparently poor diet, has disturbed sleep during the night and gastro-intestinal disturbances, and is apparently very low in mood. He has been seen by his GP, who noted Fred's feelings of lethargy and slowness in responding to questions.

The case study illustrates why a comprehensive and holistic assessment is needed to identify the needs of someone who is experiencing mental ill health. In Fred's case we can see that he has had a bereavement that seems to have led to a variety of health-related issues. He has become more socially isolated and seems to be still grieving for his wife. He is low in mood. His 'social' support seemed to have come from his animals, and their removal may have compounded his feelings of social isolation. He has neglected his own self-care needs too and appears to be using alcohol as a means of coping. He appears unconcerned about his various physical health issues.

Fred's case is not unique, and it is important for all nurses from whatever field to consider the overall health-care needs of someone with mental health problems. We might ask ourselves if the practice nurses were only interested in his leg ulcer, what other aspects of Fred's health might be missed? Likewise, if a mental health nurse was only interested in his experience of depression, what physical health issues might be missed?

Chapter summary

In this chapter, we have sought to identify the general principles and methods of assessment of people with mental health problems. We have looked at the need to avoid 'labelling' and to consider the importance of comprehensive and holistic assessments that also take into consideration lifestyle factors that may contribute to additional health burdens, while also taking into consideration the strengths that a person may have in coping with their current troubles.

Activities: brief outline answers

Activity 7.1: Communication (page 123)

It is a good idea to use open questions (that is, questions that invite more than a yes/no answer) such as 'How are you feeling today?' It is important that any questions are framed by the use of active listening, the demonstration of empathy, skilled interpersonal skills and sensitivity. Make sure you listen, and demonstrate that you are listening. Check that the person has understood your question and that have understood their reply.

Activity 7.2: Communication (page 124)

There are, of course, many ways in which you can respond to this question – and this is often suggested by the context and the person who is asking you. All too often we just say 'Fine' because that is what we think is expected. Consider, for example, the sort of information you are likely to share if this question is asked by a close confidant as opposed to your GP.

Activity 7.3: Reflection (page 126)

Comprehensive and holistic assessments focus on the whole person. They focus on the physical, psychological, social, emotional and spiritual (personal meaning) dimensions of self. In health, such assessments also consider lifestyle factors, and of increasing importance are assessments of strengths and abilities. Such assessments give a full picture of the person's needs and coping abilities.

Activity 7.4: Critical thinking (page 127)

• Blood pressure = 150/80	*Objective.*
• 'I feel I can't go on'	*Subjective.*
• Pulse = 80 bpm	*Objective.*
• Sally needs to be reminded to wash her hands before preparing food	*Functional.*
• 'I'm much happier today'	*Subjective.*
• Fred is partially sighted and needs written information in a large font size	*Functional.*

Activity 7.5: Critical thinking (page 129)

Often such assessments take into consideration not only what the person is saying but how they are saying it. For example, someone may express ideas that seem strange or they might jump between topics in a conversation, making it difficult to follow. Sometimes, someone who is low in mood might be at risk of self-harm or suicide, and an assessment of their personal safety needs to be considered. Appearance and behaviour is important to assess too – for example, does the person seem sad or anxious? Have they been neglecting their personal hygiene? Sometimes a person may seem to be engaging in a conversation with someone, but they are alone. Here, it might be necessary to ascertain if the person is hearing voices.

Activity 7.6: Decision making (page 134)

There are many possible reasons here. For example, you might not know why you have been prescribed the medication. You may have concerns over the side effects or doubt that the medication may help you. You may also have a personal preference against taking medication and prefer complementary or alternative approaches.

Further reading

Barker, P. (2004) Assessment in psychiatric and mental health nursing, 2nd edn. Cheltenham: Nelson Thornes.

This book, subtitled *In search of the whole person*, gives a clear and comprehensive overview of the assessment process, including how to conduct sensitive interviews. It also includes specific information on how to assess the needs of people with specific mental health issues.

Useful websites

www.mentalhealthrecovery.com/aboutwrap.php

Information and resources on using Wellness and Recovery Action Planning.

www.nhs.uk/healthprofile/Pages/BMI.aspx

This is the NHS Choices website, which includes information on BMI, including a helpful BMI calculator.

Chapter 8
Helping the person with mental health needs

Steven Trenoweth with Wasiim Allymamod

continued . . .

of people's needs. They must be aware of their own values and beliefs and the impact this may have on their communication with others. They must take account of the many different ways in which people communicate and how these may be influenced by ill health, disability and other factors, and be able to recognise and respond effectively when a person finds it hard to communicate.

4. All nurses must recognise when people are anxious or in distress and respond effectively, using therapeutic principles, to promote their well-being, manage personal safety and resolve conflict. They must use effective communication strategies and negotiation techniques to achieve best outcomes, respecting the dignity and human rights of all concerned. They must know when to consult a third party and how to make referrals for advocacy, mediation or arbitration.

5. All nurses must use therapeutic principles to engage, maintain and, where appropriate, disengage from professional caring relationships, and must always respect professional boundaries.

6. All nurses must take every opportunity to encourage health-promoting behaviour through education, role modelling and effective communication.

Domain 3: Nursing practice and decision-making

8. All nurses must provide educational support, facilitation skills and therapeutic nursing interventions to optimise health and well-being. They must promote self-care and management whenever possible, helping people to make choices about their health care needs, involving families and carers where appropriate, to maximise their ability to care for themselves.

Domain 4: Leadership, management and team working

2. All nurses must systematically evaluate care and ensure that they and others use the findings to help improve people's experience and care outcomes and to shape future services.

NMC Essential Skills Clusters

Cluster: Care, compassion and communication

1. As partners in the care process, people can trust a newly registered graduate nurse to provide collaborative care based on the highest standards, knowledge and competence.

By the first progression point:

1. Articulates the underpinning values of *The Code: Standards of conduct, performance and ethics for nurses and midwives* (The Code) (NMC, 2008a).

4. Shows respect for others.

5. Is able to engage with people and build caring professional relationships.

continued overleaf . . .

continued . . . •••

By the second progression point:

6. Forms appropriate and constructive professional relationships with families and other carers.

7. Uses professional support structures to learn from experience and make appropriate adjustments.

4. People can trust a newly qualified graduate nurse to engage with them and their family or carers within their cultural environments in an acceptant and anti-discriminatory manner free from harassment and exploitation.

By the first progression point:

2. Respects people's rights.

3. Adopts a principled approach to care underpinned by the code (NMC, 2008a).

5. People can trust the newly registered graduate nurse to engage with them in a warm, sensitive and compassionate way.

By the first progression point:

1. Is attentive and acts with kindness and sensitivity.

2. Takes into account people's physical and emotional responses when engaging with them.

3. Interacts with the person in a manner that is interpreted as warm, sensitive, kind and compassionate, making appropriate use of touch.

4. Provides person centred care that addresses both physical and emotional needs and preferences.

5. Evaluates ways in which own interactions affect relationships to ensure that they do not impact inappropriately on others.

6. People can trust the newly registered graduate nurse to engage therapeutically and actively listen to their needs and concerns, responding using skills that are helpful, providing information that is clear, accurate, meaningful and free from jargon.

By the first progression point:

1. Communicates effectively both orally and in writing, so that the meaning is always clear.

2. Records information accurately and clearly on the basis of observation and communication.

3. Always seeks to confirm understanding.

4. Responds in a way that confirms what a person is communicating.

5. Effectively communicates people's stated needs and wishes

Cluster: Organisational aspects of care

9. People can trust the newly registered graduate nurse to treat them as partners and work with them to make a holistic and systematic assessment of their needs; to develop a personalised plan that is based on mutual understanding and respect for their individual situation promoting health and well-being, minimising risk of harm and promoting their safety at all times.

10. People can trust the newly registered graduate nurse to deliver nursing interventions and evaluate their effectiveness against the agreed assessment and care plan.

> ### Chapter aims
>
> By the end of this chapter, you should be able to:
>
> * understand when helping should start;
> * discuss the foundations for helping;
> * outline the essential helping qualities of the nurse;
> * understand the help service users want;
> * appreciate how to work in partnership and collaboratively;
> * discuss various therapeutic strategies for helping;
> * understand the role of clinical supervision and support for the helping nurse.

Introduction

In this chapter we will explore the different methods of attempting to help the individual experiencing mental ill health along the road to recovery. If the assessment process is the starting point, then helping is the way in which we accompany someone on their journey to recovery. Sometimes such help can involve specialist care and treatment, but often it can mean taking the time to listen to and understand the person and their troubles. Sometimes helping can be practical, such as assisting the person to complete a job application or advising about welfare benefits.

It is important that the person in need of help is offered a range of care options that are timely and meet their particular needs. Such help should, wherever possible, be based on the person's expressed wishes and take into consideration all aspects of their health and social functioning. Of course, any help we offer should be evidence based – that is, help should be effective and shown to be useful to the particular individual. In this chapter we will provide an overview of the development of therapeutic relationships, and of specific therapeutic strategies such as brief interventions, motivational interviewing, problem solving, cognitive behavioural therapy and positive recovery focused interventions.

When should helping start?

The answer to this question at first seems obvious – but it is currently sparking much debate. Historically, helping has tended to start after the person experiencing mental distress is referred to specialist mental health services. Commonly, this follows a crisis in the person's life that they (and possibly their family and friends) feel unable to cope with by themselves. Care and treatment is then provided to help that person get back on their feet. This approach is therefore *reactive* – help is offered in the face of an actual or impending crisis.

But what if we want to become *proactive* – that is, offer help *before* an individual experiences mental distress? We could argue that this would change the way in which mental health care is delivered. We might see a movement away from specialist mental health services towards providing more mental health care in primary care services, such as GP surgeries. We might also see an emphasis placed on preventing mental ill health by national and community programmes that focus on well-being. We might see mental health nurses working in schools to promote coping and resilience among school children.

In reality, of course, not everyone will want proactive help, or even see the need for it, and all too often the first sign that the person is experiencing mental distress is during a crisis. We might argue, therefore, that there will always be a need for *reactive* help; nevertheless, there is much more that could be done to offer *proactive* help to those who would benefit from such support.

Foundations for helping

The essential foundation for any form of helping is the development of a therapeutic relationship (Sin and Trenoweth, 2010a). A crucial aspect of developing such a relationship is the creation of a trusting therapeutic climate within which people feel safe to talk about issues of concern to them. However, a therapeutic relationship is more than a social relationship that one might establish with a friend because it is often time limited and it is developed with the explicit intention of helping the person in need of support on the road to recovery.

Activity 8.1   *Reflection*

Essential helping qualities

Imagine that you are having problems and feel the need to talk to someone about them. What qualities would you want in that person? Why are those qualities important to you? Do you feel you have those qualities? How might you develop those qualities?

An outline answer is given at the end of the chapter.

We sometimes think that helping in mental health care is a formally therapeutic process for which education and qualifications are needed. However, when we ourselves are in need of help, we sometimes find that it is the qualities of the person we are confiding in that are the most helpful to us. Having someone to talk to that we can trust, who is genuinely interested in helping us and who can offer a listening ear when we are in need, can be very powerful in any relationship.

Sometimes our friends and families can provide us with all the help we need to deal with our troubles, but sometimes we may feel the need to talk to someone in a professional capacity. As a nurse, you may be the person that others seek to confide in. For Rogers (1951), any helping relationship needs to be underpinned by:

- empathy – understanding the service user's experiences from their perspective;
- non-judgemental warmth or unconditional positive regard – acceptance of the service user as a person who is entitled to respect and dignity; and
- genuineness – that is, an open, honest and hopeful approach reflected in being authentic, honest and truthful.

What help do service users want?

Activity 8.2   *Critical thinking*

What do *you* want?

Imagine that you are experiencing mental distress that warrants support from mental health professionals. What do you feel would be helpful to you? What sort of help do you want from mental health services?

An outline answer is given at the end of the chapter.

Service users consistently identify a number of factors as being particularly helpful in the recovery process (Nolan and Badger, 2005). These include:

- being listened to and understood;
- optimistic and hopeful attitudes from others;
- honesty in relation to prognosis and outlook;
- support, nurture and understanding from the practitioner;
- the provision of information resources and offers of treatment by the helper.

The most recent review of mental health nursing led by the Chief Nursing Officer of England (DH, 2006b) sees an essential helping role of the nurse as building and maintaining positive interpersonal relationships with service users and carers. This is often called a *therapeutic alliance* and it emphasises the partnership at the heart of the relationship (Repper and Perkins, 2003). Indeed, service users' feelings about the therapeutic relationship are also strongly associated with both their satisfaction with care and with their recovery.

Collaboration and partnership

Service users consistently state that they wish to be informed, supported and encouraged to participate and collaborate in their own care. For many this is an important part of their overall satisfaction with the help they receive. There is also a clear relationship between the extent to which people feel able to discuss their concerns and care with nurses and their subsequent agreement with treatment and care regimens. Hence, collaboration is more than 'mere' good practice; it may also help the person to become involved in their own care and to adhere to suggested treatment interventions (NICE, 2009a). Moreover, the success of any helping relationship is also likely to be influenced by the service user's view of how relevant the inter-vention is to them and how effective it is likely to be. Satisfaction with health services, however, does not rely entirely on the effectiveness of nursing care, important though this is, but also on care processes and communication with nurses. Sadly, there is evidence from a large survey of patients across a variety of clinical settings in mental health services, local primary care services, out-patient departments and emergency departments that people experiencing mental ill health do not feel involved or that they have collaborated in decisions about their own care and recovery (Healthcare Commission, 2006). Many patients in this survey cited the experiences of medical and nursing staff talking in front of them as if they were not there. There is clearly much room for improvement, and greater emphasis needs to be placed by nurses and other health-care workers on working with and alongside service users.

Look back at the case study about Sandra in Chapter 1 on page 8. Let us revisit this case with a view to considering how we might help her. It seems that Sandra sometimes breaks off contact with services – she reports that she is angry because they do not meet her needs. This might be because the sort of care that is offered is not in keeping with her personal preferences or that mental health services, she feels, are simply not listening to her or taking into account her views. This seems to be echoed by her interaction with the diabetic nurse specialist. The specialist seems to have entered into the interaction with a set of assumptions that Sandra does not agree with, and the nursing care offered seems to be based on such assumptions. As a consequence, Sandra may want the help on offer but feels unable to engage with the nurse and is therefore unable to benefit from her specialist knowledge and skills. This may have a detrimental effect on Sandra's physical health both in the short and long term.

It is very important that, wherever possible, mental health service users are involved in their own care. NICE, for example, sees mental health care as a collaborative process requiring skills in negotiating and shared decision-making – see, for example, the NICE guidelines for schizophrenia (NICE, 2009c). For nurses, working in partnership is not only good practice but also a professional requirement (see the NMC standards of competence at the start of this chapter). *The Code: standards of conduct, performance and ethics for nurses and midwives* (NMC, 2008a, p3) requires you to collaborate with those in your care by:

*   listening to the people and respond to their concerns and preferences;
*   supporting people in caring for themselves to improve and maintain their health;
*   recognising and respecting the contribution that people make to their own care and well-being;
*   making arrangements to meet people's language and communication needs;
*   sharing with people, in a way they can understand, the information they want or need to know about their health.

Therapeutic responses

There are many ways in which modern mental health care seeks to help the person experiencing mental ill health. As a nurse, you will need to reflect on your current understanding about such issues and how you may be able to respond, and then spend time considering and learning about how you might help the person who experiences mental distress or mental ill health. That is, you will need to consider the various therapeutic responses to the person with mental health issues in need of your help.

Being with

The first and most important strategy in helping is *being with* a person who experiences mental ill health. As mentioned before, the development of a collaborative therapeutic relationship between the nurse and service user is essential in the helping process. This is the foundation for nursing practice upon which therapeutic strategies should be delivered.

Being with someone is the fundamental essence of the caring process in mental health. It shows that you are concerned about the person experiencing mental distress and are sensitive to their needs. Being with someone can involve listening as people tell their stories, talking to people about their lives and experiences, participating in social activities and providing support and encouragement on the road to recovery. Service users often report that this sort of helping has been the most useful and is the most appreciated by them (Sin and Trenoweth, 2010).

Medication

Many people see the best way to help someone experiencing mental ill health as offering medication, and there are many service users who report that medication was of vital assistance to their recovery (Bennett, 2008). An in-depth overview of medication is outside the scope of this book, and you are advised to read David Healy's excellent *Psychiatric drugs explained* (Healy, 2008). However, in broad terms, the following types of medication are used in mental health care.

- *Anti-psychotics* – prescribed for people with symptoms of psychosis, particularly hallucinations and delusions. Anti-psychotic medication can be administered orally or via an injection that releases medication slowly, known as a 'depot'. Examples include the so-called first-generation drugs (such as chlorpromazine and haloperidol) and the newer atypical anti-psychotics (such as clozapine, risperidone and olanzapine).
- *Anti-depressants* – prescribed for people who are low in mood. Medication may be prescribed for people diagnosed with a moderate to severe depressive episode. Examples include the tricyclic antidepressants (such as amitriptyline and imipramine), monoamine oxidase inhibitors (MAOI) (such as phenelzine), and the newer selective serotonin reuptake inhibitors (SSRI) (such as Prozac®, Seroxat®).
- *Mood stabilisers* – prescribed for people with a diagnosis of bipolar affective disorder (sometimes referred to as manic depression). Examples include lithium and carbamazepine.
- *Anxiolytics* – prescribed for people with anxiety, often on a short-term basis. Examples include benzodiazepines, such as Valium®.

Additionally, medication may be used to manage physical dependence and withdrawal from addictive substances, such as alcohol or opiates. More recently, medication (*cholinesterase inhibitors*) has been used to control the symptoms of Alzheimer's disease (dementia) (NICE, 2006). However, these drugs appear to be effective only for a short period of time and remain very expensive.

The role of the nurse is of vital importance in the management of medication. While some nurses – termed non-medical prescribers, who have undertaken post-registration education on approved programmes – can and do prescribe medication, it is the role of all nurses to be mindful of the needs of people for whom medication has been prescribed. Certainly, it is a professional responsibility of nurses to ensure that the administration of medicines is safe and accurate, and that people in their care have given informed consent (NMC, 2008b). It is also important that nurses are able to discuss medication with service users in a clear manner, avoiding jargon and simplifying terminology wherever needed. It is vital that nurses are aware of the effect and side effects of medication (including signs of overdose) and that they treat any concerns that service users may have about their medication with respect. Nurses must also be aware of any special precautions surrounding the usage of medications (particular diets, use of alcohol and so forth) and the initial and ongoing monitoring needs of the person (regular blood tests, ECGs, and so forth). Nurses must also be mindful that some forms of medication are particularly addictive (such as the anxiolytics), and they should be able to support the service users in a wide range of non-pharmacological helping interventions, such as stress management techniques.

Psychosocial interventions

In modern mental health care, as we have seen in previous chapters, it is becoming increasingly important to help an individual's recovery in more diverse ways (Corrigan and Phelan, 2004). Of central importance is the ability to offer a range of talking therapies that give the person the opportunity to discuss and resolve problematic issues in their life. Psychosocial interventions (PSIs) is an umbrella term used to describe a broad range of therapeutic activities based on psychological and social principles, carried out in collaboration with clients, their families and others important in their social network (Sin and Trenoweth, 2010). The key characteristics of the PSI approach include:

*   conducting systematic assessments collaboratively with patients (and carers) to explore both needs and strengths;
*   educating individuals in order to improve their understanding and knowledge of health problems and mental health issues – such as the symptoms of mental distress, the links between thoughts, emotions and behaviours, treatment options and the implications that such problems may have on an individual's life, such as in their interpersonal functioning;
*   providing cognitive therapy – for example, restructuring unhelpful thinking so as view a situation differently particularly where the person feels helpless in the face of their symptoms;
*   undertaking psychological management of symptoms of mental distress, especially those that may be resistant or unresponsive to medication (for example, management of stress using relaxation techniques, mindfulness and meditation);
*   working with the families and carers in order to enhance their understanding and coping;
*   promoting medication concordance – such as ensuring informed consent, identifying and exploring negative attitudes towards medication.

All these interventions have an ultimate aim of helping the person to support themselves through increased knowledge of the illness and increased sense of empowerment (Repper and Perkins, 2003).

Brief interventions

Psychosocial interventions do not have to be a time-consuming activity, nor must we assume that therapeutic strategies have to be lengthy to be effective. As Miller and Rollnick (2002, p5) remark, *The fascinating point is that so much change occurs after so little counselling.* A wide range of studies from different countries have shown the effectiveness of *brief interventions* – so-called because these interventions are often short in duration, focusing on specific problems.

Concept summary: Solution-focused brief therapy (SFBT)

SFBT is a therapy that focuses on building solutions to identified problems (Iveson, 2002). The therapy typically last for three to five sessions and helps to marshal the person's abilities, strengths, coping strategies, past successes and resources to move the person forward out of their current troubles. It helps the person to focus on their hopes and goals rather than dwelling on present problems. An important process in SFBT is helping the person to be clear and realistic about their goals and be able to state what they wish to achieve and how. As the person moves towards their goals the therapist offers supportive encouragement. Iveson (2002) describes how a simple 0 to 10 scale can be helpful in clarifying the person's goals – where 0 is the worst possible scenario and 10 is the perfect solution to the person's current problems. SFBT tends not to dwell on the bottom end of the scale save for attempting to understand what has been helpful to the client at the present point in time. A realistic goal, Iveson suggests, is at point 7 on the scale, which allows the person to get on with their life without too much interference from the current problem. (It is unlikely perhaps that any of us would have the perfect solution to all of our problems.)

Brief interventions can take the form of a single session, a series of sessions, or even the provision of a self-help manual with little or even no personal contact. Indeed, brief interventions, *assuming they are well planned and executed, can have quite an impact, often as significant as that offered by more extensive intervention* (Duffy, 1994, p4). That is, even though an intervention may be brief, it still may make an important contribution to helping the person on the road to recovery.

For example, you may recall that we talked about screening assessments in Chapter 7. The Fast Alcohol Screen Test (FAST) (HDA, 2002) is an example of a screening assessment that offers a quick review of an individual's drinking habits. The purpose is to identify who may be at risk of using alcohol in a potentially harmful way and to subsequently offer appropriate help, information and advice based on possible hazardous patterns of alcohol use, signified by the acronym BRIEF.

- *B*enefits – the service user may be offered information about the benefits of sensible drinking.
- *R*isk factor – raising awareness of the person's current pattern of alcohol consumption and its impact on their health.
- *I*ntentions – finding out what the service users would like to do about their alcohol use (if anything), for example, to seek support in reducing intake.
- *E*mpathise – empathising and retaining a non-judgemental attitude.
- *F*eedback – giving the service user clear feedback on their levels of consumption in comparison to sensible drinking levels.

Based on the discussion of this brief intervention, referral to other specialist alcohol services may be needed or requested by the service user.

Motivational interviewing

Sometimes people experiencing mental ill health may be stuck in a particular pattern of behaviour or may be reluctant to take steps that might be helpful to their process of recovery. The person might be uncertain about the best way out of their current troubles. Sometimes they might feel that doing nothing might be for the best. Sometimes people are torn between doing something or doing nothing. This is known as *ambivalence*, and it can be a barrier to change. Ambivalence is natural and common, and is simply feeling two ways about something, being unsure as to whether to change or stay the same. The person may be weighing up the need for change with the desire to remain as they are (Miller and Rollnick, 2002).

Activity 8.3   *Reflection*

Your attempts to change

Many of us have attempted to address an aspect of our behaviour or lifestyle that we feel is problematic, and aspects of our lives we would like to change. Top of our list might be losing weight, giving up smoking or taking more exercise. We might have had some successes in addressing these problems – but we might not.

Take some time to review an unsuccessful attempt you have made to change. Why do you think you were unsuccessful?

An outline answer is given at the end of the chapter.

The focus of motivational interviewing (MI) is on helping people to explore and resolve their ambivalence about change. The approach is now widely used to assist with, for example, improving dietary intake (Vanwormer and Boucher, 2004) and weight loss (Carels et al., 2007), exercise (Bennett et al., 2007), medication concordance (Cooperman et al., 2007), diabetes (Channon et al., 2007), mental health (Arkowitz et al., 2008), chronic pain (Rau et al., 2008) and stroke rehabilitation (Watkins et al., 2007) among others.

In 2009, Miller and Rollnick defined the approach as a *person-centred method of guiding to elicit and strengthen personal motivation for change* (Miller and Rollnick, 2009, p25). The approach emphasises the importance of non-judgemental listening, empathy and four key communication skills, signified by the acronym OARS.

*   Using *O*pen questions to encourage service users to think and to talk about an issue of concern.
*   Making accurate and honest *A*ffirmations of the service user's strengths and abilities, to help build client confidence and commitment to change. (In Chapter 7 we discussed the importance of strength-oriented assessments.)
*   Listening actively and *R*eflectively to what the service user is saying, and reflecting this back to them in a way that encourages them to continue speaking while feeling understood.
*   Using *S*ummaries to allow the listener to show their interest in an individual's story and their understanding of what has been said.

Activity 8.4	Communication

OARS

Imagine you are a nurse supporting a patient who has a health issue that they would like your help in addressing. How could you use the OARS approach to discuss this issue with them?

An outline answer is given at the end of the chapter.

MI is conducted collaboratively and seeks to support the person in making the right decision for themselves. Those using this approach aim to work alongside the service user, helping them to identify concerns and to propose their own solutions rather than telling them what they should be concerned about, why they should be concerned, and what they should do about it. However, an important issue to inspire change is to help the person envision a future in which their current troubles have abated. This can be very motivating but can also appear overwhelming to the service user who may not be able to see a way out of their current troubles. Helping the person to identify their goals, exploring various options open to them, and developing an achievable and realistic plan to realise their goals (such as identifying specific short-, medium- and long-term objectives) can be very motivating.

Concept summary: stages of change

Prochaska and DiClemente considered how people change their behaviour, either with or without assistance from a therapist or nurse. Their model consists of six stages, as shown in Figure 8.1.

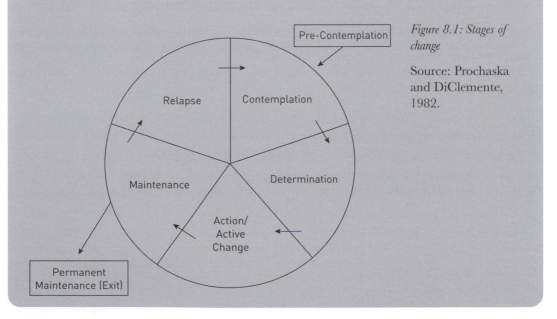

Figure 8.1: Stages of change

Source: Prochaska and DiClemente, 1982.

- Pre-contemplation (when a person is not thinking about change or is unaware of the need for change).
- Contemplation (when a person begins to think about change, but may be ambivalent).
- Determination (when a person makes the decision to change, but still with some degree of ambivalence).
- Action (the process of change).
- Maintenance (when a person continues the process of change).
- Relapse (when a person reverts to previous patterns of behaviour).

When a person no longer engages in the behaviour or is said to have permanently changed, they exit the cycle.

The 'stages of change' model is cyclical, recognising that people may go around the cycle from contemplation to relapse perhaps several times before successfully changing their behaviour. Note that the model assumes that one does not revert to a pre-contemplative stage – once one is aware of the need for change they cannot forget it. Individuals may stay in each stage for differing amounts of time, and the model suggests that providing the same help to all people is not appropriate – that specific types of interventions and help should be provided to people at different stages of change. Here, someone at the pre-contemplation stage may benefit from a conversation that raises their awareness of the risks associated with not changing their behaviour, and the benefits of changing. For example, someone recently diagnosed with diabetes may need support to raise awareness regarding the changes they may need to make to their lifestyle behaviours (particularly if they smoke, drink alcohol excessively or have a diet high in sugar and fat) and how specific treatment regimens will help to keep them healthy. This can be assisted by providing accurate information on their diagnosis and treatment, and by a subsequent discussion where any subsequent uncertainties can be clarified and the person's concerns are aired.

It is important to realise that the model suggests that interventions must be appropriate to the stage that a person is currently in – this is known as a *stage matched approach*. For example, rushing in at the pre-contemplation stage and talking about a plan to change may have little impact as the person has not yet reached the stage of deciding to change – and indeed may not even perceive the existence of a problem, let alone the need to change.

Similarly, a person at the determination stage of the model has decided to change but may lack the confidence or skills to carry out the change and to stay changed. At this stage the therapist may focus on increasing their own self-confidence in changing their behaviour. People in the action stage may benefit from skills training to help them carry out changes they have decided to make – taking more exercise, eating more healthily, managing stress better, coping with urges to smoke, and so forth. Providing someone at this stage only with information would be not be very helpful and possibly would be counterproductive, since the stage-matched approach suggests that what may be required is help and support in carrying out a planned lifestyle change. Of course, many people may just need help deciding what to do. Once they have decided, no further help may be necessary – apart, perhaps, from a mutually agreed review.

Problem-solving techniques

Sometimes a person may find it difficult to change or move on from their current troubles because they simply do not know what to do – or at least what to do for the best. It is not in keeping with a recovery approach to help someone by telling them what to do. Here, *problem-solving techniques* can be helpful to identify and explore the various options.

Problem-solving techniques assume that all problems have a solution (though the solution is not always immediately visible) and that most problems have more than one solution, and while some solutions are acceptable to the person, others may not be. It is useful therefore to generate a wide range of alternative solutions – Adair (1997) suggests a brainstorming approach to help to identify a minimum of ten possible options. Each option should be explored to identify those that are preferred, and realistic and achievable goals should be set. It is important that options are reviewed as they progress. If the goals have not been achieved, the person should be supported to reflect on why they have not been achieved and perhaps revise them accordingly. Problem-solving approaches can also be helpful in developing transferable skills, so once they are able to use problem-solving techniques they will be able to apply them to most areas of their lives, including work, personal and family life (Adair, 1997).

Cognitive behavioural therapy

Cognitive behavioural therapy (CBT) is an overarching term for a wide range of approaches that share a common focus in helping people to change problematic aspects of their thinking, feeling and behaviour. Unlike some of the other talking therapies, CBT does not focus on the causes of mental ill health but on improving a person's present state of mind. CBT usually involves weekly or fortnightly sessions with a nurse or therapist. The number of sessions required varies greatly depending on the problems that the person has, and treatment usually lasts from six weeks to six months (Simmons and Griffiths, 2009).

As with the other psychosocial interventions outlined in this chapter, CBT involves close collaboration between the nurse and service user and has proved helpful in the treatment and management of mental health conditions, including depression and schizophrenia (Gkika, 2010; Sullivan, 2010). CBT has also proved to be effective at helping people cope with, adapt to and maintain a good quality of life while living with a physical health problem and long-term conditions, not least by helping them change the way they think about and interpret their symptoms, including pain (Novy, 2004).

While there are considerable variations in the different types of CBT, these are the key elements of the approach.

- Helping the client see how CBT can offer an explanation for, and possible resolution to, the person's current troubles, including how the environment, thinking, feeling and behaving are interrelated, and how making changes to one aspect can bring about helpful changes in another.
- Helping the person to develop skills to address the identified issues, such as helping the person to recognise and change unhelpful thinking patterns, challenging unhelpful beliefs, and managing and reducing anxiety.

- Helping the person to learn from their experiences in order to prevent or reduce the risk of a relapse – including problem-solving techniques and identifying high-risk situations that may provoke a crisis.

CBT is a very flexible approach to helping people. It can be conducted by suitably trained nurses with individuals, couples or groups, or used by individuals on themselves using self-help books or computerised internet-based programmes (such as **www.beatingtheblues.co.uk/** for depression). There is much evidence that CBT is as effective as medication for the short-term treatment of many non-severe depressive and anxiety disorders. Some studies also suggest that CBT brings about a real change in how people feel about themselves and protects them from a recurrence of their problems.

Improving physical health

As mentioned in previous chapters, people with mental health problems have higher rates of physical health problems when compared to the general population (Phelan et al., 2001; DH, 2004a; DH, 2006a), including diabetes, heart problems and cancers. In addition to helping people with mental health problems to access health services, there are many ways in which the nurse can help to improve the health of a mental health client group.

As we saw in Chapter 7, people who experience mental ill health have higher rates of smoking than the general population. Smoking cessation advice and support may be an important step forward in reducing rates of mortality among mental health service users. An active lifestyle can also be an important step in preventing the development of physical health problems and has the additional benefit of contributing to an overall positive sense of physical and mental well-being. For adults the general advice is that 30 minutes of moderate-intensity physical activity at least five days a week can reduce the risk of premature death from cardiovascular disease, some cancers and significantly reduce the risk of type 2 diabetes (DH, 2004b).

Basic healthy eating advice can be an important health-promotion strategy, and information about nutrition may be helpful, assuming, of course, the person does not already know about the benefits of a healthy diet. Here, one should offer information and advice in a manner that allows the service user to make their own choices about their own diet. The information offered should reflect not only the amount that someone may be eating (perhaps too much or too little) but also the quality of food. For example, someone could be taking in excess of the guideline daily amount (GDA) of 2,000 calories per day for the typical woman and 2,500 calories per day for the typical man, but their diet may lack sufficient nutrients and fibre. The current recommendations are that everyone should eat a variety of at least five portions of fruit and vegetables each day (DH, 2004c) (a portion being 80 grams and potatoes are not included).

| Activity 8.5 | *Decision making* |

Supporting change

Imagine you are a nurse working with a patient who has a health issue that they would like your help in addressing. They might want to quit smoking, or to eat more healthily, or to take more exercise. How could you use the above strategies to help and support the person to change?

An outline answer is given at the end of the chapter.

Positive approaches

There is no doubt that mental ill health can undermine one's quality of life and subjective well-being, which compromise an individual's experience of health. You may recall that in Chapter 1 we stated that the WHO defines health as *a state of complete physical, mental and social well-being and not merely the absence of disease or infirmity* (WHO, 1946, p100). This is important as the WHO definition makes it clear that health is not the opposite of illness – that is, one does not consider oneself to be healthy simply because one does not have a disease. Moreover, it suggests that one's state of health is related to our overall holistic well-being. Hence, to promote health it is insufficient for health services to 'merely' concentrate on helping the person with a mental health problem to meet their mental health needs – we need to consider their overall well-being.

Recently, a range of positive health interventions have been developed that seem to improve health, well-being and happiness (Snyder and Lopez, 2005). It has been argued that such approaches should be in the therapeutic toolkit of all nurses (Duffy et al., 2010). As we saw in Chapter 1, recovery is a process of returning to an optimum state of wellness and the achievement of a quality of life that is personally acceptable to the individual (NIMHE, 2005a). As such, recovery is supported when:

> *Hope is encouraged, enhanced and/or maintained; Life roles with respect to work and meaningful activities are defined; Spirituality is considered; Culture is understood; Educational needs as well as those of families/significant others are identified; Socialisation needs are identified; [and when people] are supported to achieve their goals.*
> (NIMHE, 2005a, p4)

An important aspect of recovery is that of *hope*, in that a person is able to look towards the future positively and with a realistic optimism and expectation that things will be better in the long run, so the ability to inspire hope is paramount in the helping process. The hopeful person has goals that are both meaningful and desirable to them. However, the person also needs to have confidence in their ability to reach identified goals. The nurse must be enthusiastic and have the interpersonal skills to support, inspire optimism and encourage people to work towards their own personal and meaningful goals and enable the person to feel that they are being cared for and respected (Cutcliffe and Grant, 2001).

It is also important for the nurse to realise that the success of interventions is defined, at least in part, by the person receiving care. This also means that the identification of 'end goals' that individuals wish to strive for and the meaning they attach to their experiences are important (Rethink, 2005; Matthews, 2008). This is important as the nurse's evaluations of care are incomplete unless it is established how far their care has assisted the person along the road to recovery. Emphasis must be placed, therefore, on evaluating nursing care with the patient or service user and seeking their views and feedback of the success of any interventions.

An important part of the helping process is to support people to cope with life events. We have already mentioned the value of being able to solve problems, but other very important sources of support are our social networks. As nurses we need to be mindful that when faced with stressful situations, people may adopt a number of coping strategies – some of which may be ultimately more helpful than others. For example, we may temporarily avoid a stressful situation, and use tactics such as distracting ourselves. While it may be helpful in the short term, this can be unhelpful if one avoids such problems in the long term. Some people may use drugs or alcohol as a way of coping – which again is likely to be ultimately unhelpful as the person is likely to supplement their existing problem(s) with an addiction. Alternatively, we may want to take control and assume responsibility for our problems and attempt to develop realistic plans to improve our situation. We may seek out advice and support from nurses and other health-care practitioners to help us enact such strategies. That is, we may become *problem-focused*, and this approach appears to be more helpful in contributing to our overall ability to cope with difficulties (Carr, 2004).

Clinical supervision and reflection

Working with people who require our help and those who experience mental ill health requires the use of oneself and one's personal qualities and skills, along with evidence-based nursing care. It can be a demanding experience. Ultimately, nurses themselves need to feel supported in order to offer quality nursing care and treatment to people experiencing mental distress. If recovery and hope are the ultimate goals that nurses need to inspire when helping people with mental health problems, they themselves need to feel hopeful, optimistic and positive.

Clinical supervision and support from nursing colleagues are vital in that the process helps us to seek support to alleviate stress, to protect the welfare of those we care for, and to maintain personal and professional boundaries while providing us with opportunities for our personal and professional development. In addition, clinical supervision is an important mechanism by which nurses can gain constructive feedback about their work (Howatson-Jones, 2010). By reflecting on their care in a constructive, analytical and supportive way, clinical supervision helps nurses to continually improve their care and so is an important aspect of quality assurance in nursing practice.

As a student nurse, it is important that you recognise the need to be supported in caring for people and in developing helping relationships, and also to recognise the limits of your competence, that is, your ability to help (NMC, 2010b). You should seek such support when you feel it is required – it is vital that you talk to your mentor or personal tutor so that you can work through any issue that affects your ability to help.

Chapter summary

The starting point of helping is the creation of a safe, trusting therapeutic climate (built on qualities of being genuine, warm, non-judgemental and empathetic) within which people feel safe to voice their concerns. Helping, however, can also involve various interventions such as motivational interviewing, cognitive behavioural therapy, problem solving and brief interventions along with positive approaches that help the person on the road to recovery. It is vital too that the nurse is supported in their helping role. However, the main focus of any attempts at helping is that of ensuring that the service user is central to the therapeutic process and that they are able to work in partnership with the nurse.

Activities: brief outline answers

Activity 8.1: Reflection (page 146)

It is likely that you would want to chat to someone who you could trust to listen to your problems and not to dismiss them. They would not make you feel embarrassed or ashamed and you would have no problem in 'opening' up to them. You might have listed such qualities as warm, kind, supportive, encouraging and sensitive. You may also have said that you would want the person to try to understand your point of view and to show that they really were listening to you.

Activity 8.2: Critical thinking (page 147)

In addition to the essential helping qualities you outlined in Activity 8.1, you may also want some advice and support to address your current mental ill health. It is likely that you would want to feel listened to and that any treatment or nursing care offered was in keeping with your wishes. You may also have said that you would like to be offered treatment that has a good research and evidence base – that is, expert advice on interventions and care that are known to work and that have good clinical outcomes.

Activity 8.3: Reflection (page 152)

The reasons for unsuccessful attempts to change are often very individual. You might have said that you were not ready to change, or that you did not realise how difficult the change would be. Another common reason for 'relapse' is that you no longer feel that change is necessary or that the outcome of change is desirable for you. If we are giving up something that is addictive, such as cigarettes, the physiological craving can be a powerful force, and unless we are prepared for this, then our attempts to change may fail. Finally, the success of any attempts to change can be boosted by support from others, such as friends or family. Changing behaviour with another person who has a similar problem (or a group of people) can also maximise your chances of success.

Activity 8.4: Communication (page 153)

Initially, you may want to ask a broad open question to start your conversation about change. For example, you might ask the person what they would like to change about themselves. You might then ask them to talk about why they would like to change, and don't forget that here it is important to offer encouragement and support, and affirm their desire to change. Focus on the person's abilities and strengths, and help them to see the benefits of changing. Listen carefully to the person and show that you are listening. Reflect back to them what they are saying and ensure that you have clearly understood what has been said. Finally, try to summarise what the person has said and make sure that you include in your summary all the reasons why the person wants to change.

Activity 8.5: Decision making (page 157)

The starting point here is to focus on being with the person and on building a trusting relationship. In your discussions with the person you may want to ask open questions, affirm their attempts to change, reflect back to them what they have said and summarise their reasons for change. Remember that the foundations of helping include:

- being listened to and understood;
- an optimistic and hopeful attitude from others;
- honesty;
- support, nurture and understanding from practitioners;
- the provision of information resources and offers of treatment by the helper.

Helping the person also involves using a variety of interventions that have been shown to support change. Sometimes, such interventions can involve the use of medication; at other times the use of psychological or psychosocial interventions such as CBT, brief therapies or motivational interviewing may be particularly helpful. Remember that there are stages of change and that sometimes people need to consolidate a stage before moving on; for example, they might need to be clear about their reasons for change before thinking about how they might change. Make sure that you have support too and that the success of any intervention is assessed by the person who is changing.

Further reading

Gamble, C and Brennan, G (eds) (2006) Working with serious mental illness: a manual for clinical practice, 2nd edn. Edinburgh: Elsevier.

An excellent book comprising a series of chapters that highlight various aspects of helping the person experiencing mental ill health. It has become the manual for psychosocial interventions. Section 3 in particular highlights ways in which we can help the person who is experiencing mental ill health.

Useful websites

www.motivationalinterview.org/

An excellent website that contains much information on the use of motivational interviewing.

Chapter 9
Improving your own mental health

Joseph Franks

NMC Standards for Pre-registration Nursing Education

This chapter will address the following competencies:

Domain 2: Communication and interpersonal skills

6. All nurses must take every opportunity to encourage health-promoting behaviour through education, role modelling and effective communication.

Domain 3: Nursing practice and decision-making

2. All nurses must possess a broad knowledge of the structure and functions of the human body, and other relevant knowledge from the life, behavioural and social sciences as applied to health, ill health, disability, ageing and death. They must have an in-depth knowledge of common physical and mental health problems and treatments in their own field of practice, including co-morbidity and physiological and psychological vulnerability.

7. All nurses must be able to recognise and interpret signs of normal and deteriorating mental and physical health and respond promptly to maintain or improve the health and comfort of the service user, acting to keep them and others safe.

8. All nurses must provide educational support, facilitation skills and therapeutic nursing interventions to optimise health and well-being. They must promote self-care and management whenever possible, helping people to make choices about their health care needs, involving families and carers where appropriate, to maximise their ability to care for themselves.

10. All nurses must evaluate their care to improve clinical decision-making, quality and outcomes, using a range of methods, amending the plan of care, where necessary, and communicating changes to others.

Domain 4: Leadership, management and team working

4. All nurses must be self-aware and recognise how their own values, principles and assumptions may affect their practice. They must maintain their own personal and professional development, learning from experience, through supervision, feedback, reflection and evaluation.

NMC Essential Skills Clusters

This chapter will address the following ESCs:

Cluster: Care, compassion and communication

1. As partners in the care process, people can trust a newly registered graduate nurse to provide collaborative care based on the highest standards, knowledge and competence.

By the first progression point:

1. Articulates the underpinning values of *The code: standards of conduct, performance and ethics for nurses and midwives* (the code) (NMC, 2008a).
2. Works within limitations of the role and recognises own level of competence.
3. Promotes a professional image.
4. Shows respect for others.
5. Is able to engage with people and build caring professional relationships.

By the second progression point:

6. Forms appropriate and constructive professional relationships with families and other carers.
7. Uses professional support structures to learn from experience and make appropriate adjustments.

By entry to the register:

8. Demonstrates clinical confidence through sound knowledge, skills and understanding relevant to field.
9. Is self aware and self confident, knows own limitations and is able to take appropriate action.
10. Acts as a role model in promoting a professional image.
11. Acts as a role model in developing trusting relationships, within professional boundaries.
12. Recognises and acts to overcome barriers in developing effective relationships with service users and carers.

Chapter aims

By the end of this chapter, you should be able to:

- define health and understand its historical and contemporary context;
- describe concepts of holism when thinking of health;
- demonstrate an understanding of stress and its implications for health;
- explore stress and the individual's vulnerability to stress;
- discuss adaptive and maladaptive coping strategies;
- understand the concept of Wellness Recovery Action Planning (WRAP).

Introduction

> ### Case study
>
> *Jim is a student nurse on his first practice learning experience; in the week leading up to it he has become increasingly nervous and anxious. On the first day Jim finds the environment busy, bewildering and stressful. At the end of the first shift he is unhappy with the whole experience and treats himself to a bottle of wine, thinking it will help him relax. After a bad night's sleep he goes back to work nervous, anxious and tired. The day starts badly and just gets worse, which adds to Jim's stress; he feels he can't complete this practice learning opportunity as he feels inadequate and physically ill. He wonders how all the other staff appear to deal with the pressure.*

In this chapter we will first examine and define concepts of health and how the historical context of health and well-being has affected contemporary approaches towards the treatment of mental health. This will be followed by examining the idea of holism when treating the patient with mental health difficulties by appreciating how biological, psychological, social, spiritual and emotional aspects of the individual encompass the idea of holism. We will then examine the concept of stress as a major factor that can affect health and be determined by our individual attributes. You will be encouraged to relate the impact of stress to your own experiences and how this may also contribute to your health and that of the patient while thinking of why certain individuals may be vulnerable to stress; this will be framed within a stress vulnerability model. You will also be guided towards ideas for coping and will be encouraged to reflect on your own coping strategies for stress; we will find out whether coping is adaptive or maladaptive. We will find out how to improve coping strategies and how this impacts on your own mental health and that of patients. The chapter will conclude by introducing the reader to the Wellness Recovery Action Plan or WRAP (Copeland, 1997). The WRAP is based on the study of coping and wellness for people who have experienced mental health challenges. It centres on self-help, recovery and long-term stability.

Historical and contemporary context of health

What is health and how do we define it? The English word 'health' is derived from an Old English word *hale*, which means simply wholeness, being whole, sound or well (Nordqvist, 2009). If we consider this definition of health, we may conclude that it implies that wholeness or being whole occurs when the mind and body are working together in harmony. We may further infer from this definition that to produce a state of wellness we should consider the mind and body as connected and not as two entities to be treated separately. The idea that the way people feel in their minds can influence the way they feel in their bodies, or vice versa, and the idea that of mind and body are interconnected and working in tandem have existed for centuries. The classical Greek philosopher Plato (428/427 BC–348/347 BC) advocated the importance of physical exercise for developing the mind, and Hippocrates (460 BC–370 BC), considered to be the founding father of Western medicine, also held the belief that the body must be treated as a whole and not just as a series of parts. He is known to have stated: *It is better to know the man who has the disease than the disease the man has.* The later Greco-Romans incorporated these ideas into their culture, having as their motto *mens sana in corpora sano*, a sane mind in a sane body. When looking back over time we can see that the idea of holism or of mind and body working together when approaching health and well-being was considered central to the philosophies of medicine. This is certainly true during and beyond the Greco-Roman period. So when and how did this seemingly artificial distinction arise in our consciousness and when did we begin to lose these fundamental holistic concepts when approaching mind, body and health? Descartes (1596–1650) is thought by many to be responsible for the erosion of these ideas. Descartes was a French philosopher, mathematician and physicist who advocated the separation of the body and mind. This is known as Descartes dualism. Descartes' philosophy viewed the body in reductionist terms; the body was seen as a machine, and any disorders were due to the malfunctioning of individual parts of the body, therefore separating and deconstructing the body from the mind. It was from this time onwards that we began to lose the concept of holism, and with this came the rise and eventual dominance of the biomedical approach to mental health. It is only fairly recently that the approach towards the treatment of mental health has again begun to move forwards towards the idea of holism or of a holistic view of mental health.

So what are the contemporary definitions of health and how do these relate to health-care practice today? The WHO (1946) defined health as a *state of complete physical, mental and social well-being and not merely the absence of disease or infirmity.* This is an interesting definition as it recognises health as comprising more than just the absence or presence of disease; it takes a holistic approach to health and the determinants of health. However, since this definition, health care has appeared to remain focused on the disease concepts of health, although modern health-care services are beginning to recognise and utilise holistic approaches to health. When approaching the care and treatment of those with poor health, what determinants of health should be accounted for to effectively deliver treatments or interventions? The Department of Health (1999a) reported that poor health springs from a range of wider community factors, including poverty, low wages, unemployment, poor education, substandard housing, crime and disorder and a polluted environment. Determinants of health can also be considered as including broad domains that may include the following.

- Income and social status – higher income and social status are linked to better health; the greater the gap between the richest and poorest people, the greater the differences in health.
- Education – low education levels are linked with poor health, more stress and lower self-confidence.
- Physical environment – safe water and clean air, healthy workplaces, safe houses, communities and roads all contribute to good health.
- Employment and working conditions – people in employment are healthier, particularly those who have more control over their working conditions.
- Social support networks – greater support from families, friends and communities is linked to better health.

- Culture – customs and traditions, and the beliefs of the family and community all affect health.
- Genetics – inheritance plays a part in determining lifespan, healthiness and the likelihood of developing certain illnesses.
- Personal behaviour and coping skills – balanced eating, keeping active, smoking, drinking, and how we deal with life's stresses and challenges all affect health.
- Health services – access and use of services that prevent and treat disease influences health.
- Gender – Men and women suffer from different types of diseases at different ages.

(WHO, 2011)

Case study

Jayne is a newly qualified nurse who works on an inpatient unit for older adults with a variety of health needs. A new patient called Dorothy is admitted to the unit, and at first glance at the nursing notes the reason appears to be to treat persistent leg ulcers that refuse to heal. After Jayne speaks with Dorothy and the community nurse a different picture of Dorothy's overall health begins to emerge.

Dorothy lives alone in the community with a weekly visit from the community nurse who dresses and treats Dorothy's leg ulcers. The community nurse reports that as well as the obvious physical presentation she has other concerns regarding Dorothy. It seems that since Dorothy's husband passed away the house has been neglected and is in a rather squalid state with unwashed crockery, rubbish and laundry strewn about the house. Dorothy also keeps cats that have been using different parts of the house as a toilet, and this compounds the general hygiene concerns. Dorothy neglects to maintain a healthy diet and rarely leaves the house to buy anything other than the bare essentials, and although she is entitled to certain state benefits, she is not in receipt of these. Dorothy doesn't work, has lost contact with her friends and rarely sees her family.

Jayne now has a fuller picture of Dorothy's circumstances and begins to see that the leg ulcers are just a small but interlinked aspect of Dorothy's overall health. Without addressing Dorothy's wider health needs the leg ulcers are unlikely to heal as Jayne realises that all of these health issues interact, are connected and impact on one another.

Activity 9.1   *Reflection*

Put yourself in Jayne's position and reflect upon what you would do if faced with this situation. What wider determinants of health would you consider when thinking about Dorothy and her care? Once you have identified these, how would you go about addressing those health determinants? How would you coordinate this and with whom?

An outline answer is given at the end of the chapter.

Holism and health

So how does this separation of mind and body translate into mental health care today? Despite the ideas of holism or holistic care most lay people and, unfortunately, many health-care professionals still view disorders of the mind as separate from the body. This is further compounded by the division of health-care provision into these two distinct camps, which only reinforces this assumption of a body and mind distinction. The treatment of those with mental health problems within health care remains distinct from those with other illnesses; although efforts have been made to bridge this gap there still remains the problem of inequality within the delivery of health care. One such problem when treating those with mental health problems is that of their physical health. Physical health is often overlooked or does not receive the appropriate attention it requires, as the emphasis on treatment remains focused on the mind (DH, 2006b). This focus of attention has also sidelined social and spiritual aspects of care when treating patients, but the lack of attention to physical health is of particular concern. Those suffering from severe mental illness are more likely to die on average ten years earlier when compared with the rest of the population. This is due to a variety of reasons such as the undesirable side effects of anti-psychotic medication, smoking, lack of exercise and weight gain (DRC, 2006). Increasingly, this issue has gained attention. Government policy has recognised that attending to the physical health needs of people with **serious mental illness** (SMI) is associated with improvements in both mental and physical health, particularly in terms of patients' improved self-esteem (DH, 2006a). Despite advancements in the attention paid to the physical health needs of those with SMI and the recognition that good physical health can enhance mental health, these inequalities still exist in this group of people when compared to the general population.

Activity 9.2	Reflection

Think about a time when you were faced with an impending exam, deadline for an essay, first flight, first day at university or meeting new people, etc. How did this make you feel and think? Consider how you felt mentally and physically – you may have felt nervous or anxious. Now pause for a moment and think of the physical sensations you experienced. Maybe you noticed your heart racing, your palms sweating, or perhaps you spent more time on the toilet than normal. Make a note of how you felt.

An outline answer is given at the end of the chapter.

What you noted down in the activity are examples of how you feel mentally (anxious, nervous, etc) affects the way you feel physically. These are just some of the obvious ways in which your mind and body are linked. Now think about what causes you to feel nervous and anxious and give you those physical sensations. It is the stress caused by the impending exam, essay or first day at university that triggers those thoughts and feelings.

There are many other ways in which we experience this connection between mind and body. For example, how do you feel when you have the flu or a heavy cold? As well as the physical symptoms, your mood may be low, you may be fed up that you feel so ill you cannot go out, see your friends, catch up with work or go to university. Now think of how a person might feel if they have a debilitating disease such as cancer or HIV. They will not just be suffering with the physical symptoms of this disease; they will possibly have a range of psychological and emotional difficulties such as anxiety about the future, depression because they feel hopeless and perhaps they feel despairing and suicidal. There is a balance between good physical health/positive well-being and mental health. You cannot have one without the other. The science of this vital link is called **psychoneuroimmunology**.

If we think about improving our own mental health or that of others, the focus must not be on either the body or the mind but on the whole. When we take a holistic approach to mental health and accept the notion that neither mind nor body develops illness – only *people* develop illnesses – we can then begin to think about the individual. When thinking of the individual or the whole person this should include the wider interactions between biological, psychological, social, spiritual and emotional aspects of their and our own lives, particularly when considering the improvement of mental health and well-being.

How do we define well-being and mental health?

The WHO (2010) defines good mental health as a state of well-being in which the individual realises his or her own abilities, can cope with the normal stresses of life, can work productively and fruitfully, and is able to make a contribution to his or her community. So it is more than just the absence of mental illness. In this definition it is important to note the emphasis on *coping with the normal stresses of life*, as stress can be a major contributing factor to the development of mental ill health, particularly when we lose or have limited capacity to cope with stress. Well-being as defined by the DH (2009a) is seen as a positive state of mind and body, feeling safe and able to cope, with a sense of connection with people, communities and the wider environment. These two definitions are separate but interconnected, with positive well-being acting as a buffer to stress and developing mental health problems.

Improving your own mental health

Many of us can have symptoms of mental distress but would not recognise these symptoms as of clinical significance: indeed, you can have symptoms of mental distress without these symptoms ever developing into what would be recognised clinically as a mental health problem. For both clinical and non-clinical groups, strategies to improve mental health and well-being would remain broadly similar. Modest improvements in mental health between either group can bring worthwhile improvements in their overall quality of life. Improvements in mental health, even small ones, can have a positive impact on physical health, productivity and quality of life (NIMHE, 2005a).

So what can you do to improve or protect your own mental health? The National Institute for Mental Health in England (NIMHE, 2005a) suggests strategies drawn from research into what people with mental health problems find helpful with regard to protecting their mental health. NIMHE calls these strategies the 'five fruit and veg' of mental health help that will help protect the mental health of everyone, whether or not they have symptoms of mental distress. They include:

- keeping physically active;
- eating well;
- drinking in moderation;
- valuing yourself and others;
- talking about your feelings;
- keeping in touch with friends and loved ones;
- caring for others;
- getting involved and making a contribution;
- learning new skills;
- doing something creative;
- taking a break;
- asking for help.

The Foresight Mental Capital and Well-being Project (2008) was commissioned by the UK Government Office for Science to look at how best to achieve mental development and mental well-being for everyone in the UK today and in later years. This is a comprehensive project that draws together the best available evidence from around the world and is divided into five broad areas: learning through life; mental health; well-being; and work and learning difficulties.

Although a valuable and comprehensive document, it lacked recommendations for what could be built into day-to-day living to improve mental well-being. So in 2008, the Foresight Mental Capital and Well-being Project commissioned the New Economics Foundation to do just that – review the work of over 400 scientists from across the world with the aim of identifying a set of evidence-based actions to improve well-being that individuals would be encouraged to integrate into their daily lives. *Five Ways to Well-being* (Aked et al., 2008) drew upon the best evidence and selected strategies that did not rely on external resources, such as money, and that were user friendly and accessible, so that no matter what background, economic status or social class you came from, the Five Ways could be easily applied. We shall explore these Five Ways and the evidence that supports them. You will also be invited to consider nutrition as an additional but important factor that contributes to overall health and well-being. It is not included in the Five Ways as it is considered reliant on external factors, but it remains an important subject area with regard to health and well-being.

Connect

> *Connect with the people around you. With family, friends, colleagues and neighbours. At home, work, school or in your local community. Think of these as the cornerstones of your life and invest time in developing them. Building these connections will support and enrich you every day.*
> (Aked et al., 2008, p5)

What does the above statement mean when thinking of your own well-being and improving your own and the patient's mental health? We have seen in Chapter 1 that social models of mental distress play a major role in influencing mental health, especially among those who suffer with SMI. When thinking of holism and the biological, social and psychological aspects of the whole person, then to 'connect' would fall under the social aspect of this and will impact on the psychological through a sense of improved well-being or improved mental health. So it would make sense to assume that social models of mental distress can be inverted to apply to improving the mental health and well-being of ourselves. Research has shown that happy people have stronger social relationships than less happy people (Diener and Seligman, 2002). If we can apply the ability to 'connect' successfully to our own lives and understand what factors contribute to an improved sense of well-being, then we can be confident when approaching and helping patients towards recovery, particularly when considering the social aspects of mental health and well-being. To 'connect' can also be considered in the broader terms 'social inclusion' versus 'social exclusion'. Beck et al. (1997) defined social inclusion as *the extent to which citizens are able to participate in the social and economic life of their communities under conditions that enhance their well-being and individual potential.* Huxley and Thornicroft (2003) argued that this could be achieved by enabling people to develop or rejoin their leisure, friendship and work communities. It is also important to consider why people with an SMI suffer a greater degree of social exclusion than those without an SMI; patients with an SMI are generally faced with greater adversity in terms of social exclusion/ inclusion through stigma, lack of community tolerance, etc. Those with a long-term SMI are among the most excluded in society (Social Exclusion Unit, 2004).

Social relationships are essential for promoting well-being and acting as a protective factor against developing mental health problems. Good social networks also promote a sense of belonging and well-being (Morrow, 2001),

Be active

Go for a walk or run. Step outside. Cycle, play a game, garden, dance. Exercising makes you feel good. Most importantly, discover a physical activity you enjoy; one that suits your level of mobility and fitness.
(Aked et al., 2008, p6)

The importance of exercise for improving physical health is well known. If we think back to earlier in the chapter and how good physical health can affect positive outcomes with mental health, then it is not surprising to see that being active can also improve your sense of well-being. If we pause to think of holism and the biological, psychological and social aspects of the whole person, we can frame physical activity as influencing the biological and the psychological aspects of this model. If we engage in physical activity within groups, then you can also positively influence the social. Activity is, in fact, beneficial to the individual on all of these areas. Physical activity does not necessarily have to be vigorous to produce feelings of well-being. The promotion of the importance of exercise has seen a number of policies developed, which have called for regular, moderate intensity activity on most days of the week, with recommendations tailored to individual needs, such as those of young people, adults, older adults or those with certain medical conditions (Department of Health and Human Services and Centres for Disease Control and Prevention, 1996; DH, 2004b). Some particular benefits of longer-term or habitual physical activity have also been reported; these include a reduction in anxiety and depression, improved mood and sleep, improved ability to deal with stress and improved cognitive function.

While the evidence base for exercise and well-being is still developing, it appears that general agreement has emerged about the efficacy of exercise for well-being. It is likely to be essential for all age groups, and if physical activity, such as walking, is enjoyed in groups or with friends, then social interaction will be encouraged, improving the ability to connect.

Take notice

Be curious. Catch sight of the beautiful. Remark on the unusual. Notice the changing seasons. Savour the moment, whether you are on a train, eating lunch or talking to friends. Be aware of the world around you and what you are feeling. Reflecting on your experiences will help you appreciate what matters to you.
(Aked et al., 2008, p8)

How often do you pause or take a moment to look up and take in the sunset, a full moon or the colours in the trees as the seasons pass? Do you stop and notice the changing seasons? How aware are you of the natural world around you? Unfortunately our busy lives often consist of rushing around from one task to the next – perhaps dropping children off at school and then rushing to work or college, only to do it again the following day. In between, you probably find that you are thinking about the next task or planning the day or week ahead. It takes but a moment to look up and be aware of the world around you and to remain in that moment. When you see the sun setting from the train window or the sunlight dancing on the reds and yellows of the autumn colours in the trees, do you stop to take notice and consciously notice the sensations that these sights engender? Or do you merely notice, hurry on and not give it a second thought?

Much research has looked at how changes in behaviour may act as a means to improving our sense of well-being. One such study by Fredrickson (2003) concluded that being aware of what is taking place in the present directly enhances well-being (cited by Aked et al., 2008). When you consciously stop and take note of the world around you, take note and be aware of your sensations, thoughts and feelings, it has been shown to enhance feelings of well-being. These ideas are known as **mindfulness** and can also be thought of as *the state of being attentive to and aware of what is taking place in the present* or *the clear and single-minded awareness of what actually happens to us and in us at the successive moments of perception* (Nyanaponika, 1972). The concept of mindfulness has its roots in Buddhism, and a wealth of literature and evidence is now available that cites its effectiveness when its use is promoted among those with mental health problems. This is particularly the case with cognitive behavioural therapy, which is increasingly integrating mindfulness within its approaches to treatment.

Keep learning

Try something new. Rediscover an old interest. Sign up for that course. Take on a different responsibility at work. Fix a bike. Learn to play an instrument or how to cook your favourite food. Set a challenge you will enjoy achieving. Learning new things will make you more confident, as well as being fun to do.
(Aked et al., 2008, p9)

How often do you think about signing up for a new course, reigniting an old hobby or learning a new skill? Like many of us, you may think about it and perhaps put it off until later, or you might decide it is not the right time. How do you feel when you do learn a new skill, complete an academic course or engage in that long-forgotten hobby? Does it give you a sense of accomplishment, boost your confidence and self-esteem and increase your sense of well-being? The evidence suggests that these are examples of how you would feel when you achieve these goals. Schuller et al. (2002) confirm this by stating that the most fundamental benefit from learning of every kind is a growth in self-confidence. Sabates and Hammond (2008) add to this by concluding that participation in learning increases self-confidence and self-esteem. Furthermore, goal setting, which is particularly associated with adult learning, has also been shown to have a strong correlation with higher levels of well-being *when the goals are self generated and congruent with personal values* (Huppert, 2008). So it appears that learning and goal setting can have a positive impact on your well-being, but it is important to note from the literature that learning and goal setting that is intrinsic (from within) produce feelings of well-being, while extrinsic pressures to learn (for example, being required by your employer) can reduce your motivation to achieve.

Give

Do something nice for a friend, or a stranger. Thank someone. Smile. Volunteer your time. Join a community group. Look out, as well as in. Seeing yourself, and your happiness, linked to the wider community can be incredibly rewarding and will create connections with the people around you.
(Aked et al., 2008, p10)

For hundreds of years, most people lived in the place they were born, surrounded by their family or clan. They knew everyone and belonged to a tightly knit group. The modern Western world over the years has witnessed the fragmentation of the extended family unit and the breakdown of the community. There is a sense among some that the decline in community walks hand in hand with the rise of **individualism**. The proportion of people who know their neighbours has dropped over the years, with some saying this has contributed to the loss of a feeling of community. It is now recognised that community involvement and being part of a community can have a positive impact on our sense of well-being. It is well known that we are social animals; our human nature dictates a need for mutual and social cooperation. The **neurosciences** provide evidence for this by demonstrating that mutual cooperation is associated with enhanced neuronal response in reward areas of the brain, which indicates that social cooperation is intrinsically rewarding (Rilling et al., 2007). To put this in layman's terms, when you engage in mutual social cooperation, certain parts of the reward systems of your brain are activated, which in turn trigger a sense of well-being. Appropriate stimulation of this reward system, particularly in early life, contributes to gains in cognitive and social functioning critical for the development of well-being (Aked et al., 2008). Huppert (2008) reports in the Foresight Mental Capital and Well-being Project that feelings of happiness and life satisfaction have been strongly associated with active participation in social and community life. Lyubomirsky et al. (2005) reports in their study of happiness that the act of helping others has also been shown to improve feelings of well-being. His studies have shown that committing an act of kindness once a week over a six-week period has been associated with an increase in well-being (cited by Aked et al., 2008).

Case study

John is a community psychiatric nurse and visits a new patient called Jim who has just been allocated as part of his case load. After the visit John writes in Jim's case notes the following.

Jim suffers with depression and lives alone in his flat. He doesn't have a job and spends most of his time sitting in his flat. The local area is run down although a short bus ride would give him access to local

continued overleaf . . .

continued . . . . •••

amenities, parks, shops, etc. Jim has little contact with his family or neighbours although his family live locally. Jim used to visit the local Roman Catholic Church for mass but he has also stopped doing this. The only real contact he has is with professionals from the community mental health team. He rarely leaves the flat, choosing to sit in front of the TV with the curtains closed, though he does occasionally visit a nearby newsagent to buy cigarettes or essential items. As a result Jim is socially isolated, has little interaction with his community and limited opportunity to do so, as he isolates himself. His diet is poor, and this in part has led to poor physical health. Jim wants to improve his situation and is fed up with feeling depressed.'

Activity 9.3   *Reflection*

Now think about what you have read in this chapter so far. How would you feel if you were in a similar situation to Jim? What would you do to improve your situation? Think about what is important to you in your life and how you could apply these things to Jim to improve his situation. Take into consideration the mind–body connection, holism, biological, social, psychological and spiritual domains of holism. As John, the CPN, what would you discuss with Jim and encourage him to do? How would you explain this to Jim, and what reasons would you give Jim for changing his behaviour?

Some suggestions are given in the brief outline answers at the end of the chapter.

The Five Ways make recommendations for what we can add to our day-to-day routine to improve well-being, reduce stress and protect against developing mental health difficulties. Nutrition is another important factor to consider when thinking of mental health, and we examine this next before moving on to stress, and strategies for coping with stress and stressful situations.

Nutrition

When thinking of nutrition and physical health we can recognise how a poor diet can impact on us physically. For example, a high salt intake affects our blood pressure, high saturated fat affects cholesterol levels, and a lack of fruit and vegetables impacts the potential for developing cancer and cardiovascular diseases. How often do you think of the impact of your diet on your mental health? If you think about how poor nutrition affects physical health, should the same not apply to your mental health? Over the years a growing body of evidence has been developing that demonstrates a link between our diets and our mental health; after all, we are in essence what we eat. Considering this, we will briefly discuss the brain and some of its biology, and look at how diet can affect this and the impact on our mental health. The function of the brain and its effect on our mental health is a topic too vast to cover in this chapter and as a topic occupies many books in its own right, so a brief overview will be given to enable the reader to place this subject in context when considering diet and mental health.

If we think for a moment how a poor diet or poor nutrition can affect our bodies and its individual organs, it should come as no surprise to suppose that the same will be the case for the brain, which is the largest organ in the body. The brain is an enormously complex system and is the most complex organ within the human body. Science is only now beginning to understand the brain; much is still unknown and much is yet to be discovered. The brain is the largest organ in our bodies and is made up of billions of nerve cells called **neurons**. Neurons make up different pathways within the brain with the neurons communicating with each other through complex electrical and chemical messages. The medium that the neurons use to communicate between one another are called **neurotransmitters**, and these are made up of nutrients. This communication allows the brain to function and in turn regulates such things as our mood, sleep, movement and pain relief.

The key to the neurons' ability to communicate effectively is the cell membranes' fluidity and functionality, which allows the cell membrane to change shape. This flexibility is attributed to the makeup of the brain, which is comprised of unsaturated fatty acids, which are the most flexible type of fat (Van de Weyer, 2005). These fatty acids, specifically omega 3 and omega 6, are acquired through our diet. Omega 3 is predominantly found in fish and omega 6 is predominantly found in seed oils (sunflower and soybean); the lack of omega 3 in Western diets is increasingly implicated in mental illness and a lack of functionality and fluidity in the cell membrane of the neuron. Interestingly, the modern Western diet has evolved into a meat and saturated-fat rich diet, with falling consumption of fresh vegetables and fish, but a large rise in the consumption of seed oils. This shift away from food sources rich in omega 3 in the Western diet parallels the rise in mental illnesses seen in the last century (Hallahand and Garland, 2005).

Neurotransmitters are made from chemical **precursors** which are generally **proteins** or **amino acids**. Some amino acids can be made in the body, but essential amino acids have to be obtained from the diet. Some of these essential amino acids include **leucine**, **phenylalanine**, **lysine** and **tryptophan** and are precursors or forerunners of neurotransmitters. If our diet does not include enough of these amino acids, then theoretically this could create communication problems between the neurons (Van de Weyer, 2005). To convert precursors into neurotransmitters a number of different enzymes, minerals and vitamins have to be present. Tryptophan as a chemical precursor is implicated in the manufacture of serotonin, the neurotransmitter concerned with the regulation of mood. For those who are prone to depression the observation has been made that by manipulating the tryptophan content of their diet, a hastening of depressed mood can be made (Delgado et al., 1990).

The connection between diet, mental health, mental illness and well-being cannot be overlooked; not only is a balanced diet a useful protective buffer to developing a mental illness, but it is also important as a factor to be considered when taking a holistic approach to the treatment of mental illness.

For a comprehensive and detailed link between nutrition and mental health, see 'Useful websites' at the end of the chapter.

Stress and implications for health

As every nursing student knows, stress is an inevitable fact of modern life. There are two broad categories: ambient stress and life event stress. Ambient stress is seen as the day-to-day 'hassles' of life such as unexpected bills, unsatisfying job prospects, meeting deadlines for essays or the prospect of a long lecture at university. Perhaps you have children to take to school before attending university, money to find to pay for that unexpected council tax bill or a student bursary that is too small? All of these everyday worries can be classed as ambient or background stress. Individuals are affected by these stresses in varying degrees, but most manage to maintain reasonable health and functioning under these stressful conditions (Folkman, 1992). The second categories of stress are major life events. These events are recognised by most people as highly stressful. They occur to most people at some points in their lives, and include bereavement, divorce, serious financial strain, unemployment and serious illness. It is also important to note that stress can also include positive life events (such as marriage or job promotion). The list for either is not exhaustive and is dependent on the individual, their perceived ability to cope and the context in which stress is experienced.

Exposure to excessive or chronic stress can have a number of physical and psychological effects, some of which are recognised as anxiety, depression, agitation, insomnia, irritability, low motivation, anger, frustration, poor concentration, back pain, migraine and difficulties in decision making. Stress is also a major factor implicated in the development of mental health problems, which we will examine later in this chapter.

Physiology of stress

So what is the biology of stress and how does it affect you physically? When your body is faced with a perceived stressful situation it prepares itself to fight or flee. This 'fight or flight response' is said to be an evolutionary defence mechanism from a time when mankind still faced natural predators. Your body prepares for this fight or flight response by releasing a number of hormones such as **adrenaline** and **cortisol**, which causes common symptoms of stress: sweating, a rise in blood pressure and increased heart rate. Cortisol is also the hormone responsible for other biological functions such as glucose metabolism, regulation of blood pressure, insulin levels, immune function and inflammatory responses. These hormones prepare your body for either fight or flight, or give your body a burst of energy or strength in preparation to deal with a perceived threat. Stressful situations in the modern world are more often than not situations where we do not find ourselves faced by a predator so we have no opportunity to fight or flee; we find that the response is activated through stress at university, impending exams and starting a new clinical learning experience and so on. In these situations, after the stressful event has passed your body has a chance to relax or return to normal functioning. It is only when you are faced with chronic or persistent stressful situations that you will see the emergence of physical and psychological problems.

With chronic or recurring stress the hormone levels do not have the chance to return to normal, and this can result in persistently high levels of stress hormone; it is then that you see the emergence of stress-related health problems. Some common health problems related to chronic and prolonged stress are persistently high blood pressure, heart disease, diabetes, stroke and memory loss. The emergence of these stress-induced problems, as noted previously, can be mediated by the individual's susceptibility to these stressors or their vulnerability to stress. Stress can also cause psychological problems and, in those that are vulnerable, the development of mental health problems. For individuals with pre-existing serious mental illnesses, stress can be a major contributing factor to relapse into an episode of illness. Excessive stress is also responsible for causing psychological problems, which can either be somatic complaints such as body aches and pain or sleeplessness, or psychological disturbances such as anxiety, self-medicating or eating disorders and emotional problems (Freidmen and Silver, 2007). The most commonly reported symptoms of chronic stress include insomnia, frequent headaches, personality changes, irritability, anxiety and depression. Stress can lead to concentration problems, low sexual desire or libido, performance anxiety, excessive worry or guilt, nervousness, anger, frustration, hostility, mood swings, changes in appetite, racing thoughts, obsessive-compulsive behaviours and social withdrawal.

Vulnerability to stress

What can make one person particularly vulnerable to stress and another person resilient to its effects? Factors that are thought to play a role here include major life events, social isolation, physical diseases, genetic dispositions, early life experiences and personality traits. We have discussed the role that important life events, social isolation and physical ill health can play with regard to stress and health, but what about your personality, genetics and early life events? Genetics are thought to play a role when determining how vulnerable we are to stress, although they are thought to be only part of the picture – complex interactions between genetics and environmental stressors are involved, and when we experience enough stress, certain genes are thought to express themselves. Evidence from family studies, particularly studies involving twins, seems to show a strong genetic element (Horrobin, 2001). So if you are particularly prone to stress or have a low genetic vulnerability, relatively small amounts might be enough to push you into an episode of physical or mental distress. Early life events tend to be childhood trauma that can leave a lasting effect on our ability to cope with stress, particularly if these experiences are left unresolved. Examples include sexual and physical abuse, neglect, witnessing acts of violence or abuse and chronic maltreatment. A clear link between childhood abuse, maltreatment and the future development of mental health problems in adulthood has been demonstrated in a number of studies (e.g. Spataro et al., 2004).

Personality

Another aspect of an individual's vulnerability to stress that can play a contributing factor is that of personality. Personality can either increase or decrease your vulnerability to stress. The correlations between personality traits and health are too numerous and complex to cover in their entirety within this chapter. An overview will be given of some of the research findings in this field before examining stress, personality traits and adaptive and maladaptive coping with regard to stress.

Trait theories

Trait theories of personality are one of the major theoretical areas within the study of personality. Trait theory states that personality traits remain relatively stable over time, that traits differ among individuals and that behaviour is influenced by these traits. Traits are seen as functioning along a continuum with individuals falling anywhere within this continuum. Within trait theory several models exist, with one model widely acknowledged and accepted by personality psychologists. This model is nicknamed the 'Big Five' and contains the following dimensions of personality.

1. *Openness or Intellect*: characteristics of this trait are imagination, insight, an interest in variety and independence. Those who are high in this trait also tend to have a broad range of interests. Those who are low in this trait or closed tend to have narrow common experiences and prefer familiarity over the novel.
2. *Conscientiousness*: common for this trait is the propensity to be careful, organised, goal directed and aware of detail. Those who score low in this trait tend to be easy going and careless and unreliable.
3. *Extraversion*: this trait may include a propensity to be outgoing, fun loving, sociable and assertive. Those who score low in this trait or introverts tend to be quiet, low key and deliberate.
4. *Agreeableness*: the tendency to be compassionate, trusting, kind and affectionate is characteristic of this trait. Those who score low in this trait or are disagreeable tend to display self-interest above getting along with others.
5. *Neuroticism or Emotional Stability*: common within this trait is the propensity to be anxious, irritable, sad and vulnerable to stress. High scorers are more likely to interpret minor hassles in life as hopelessly difficult. Those who score low in this trait tend to be calm, emotionally stable and free from continual negative feelings.

The Big Five trait theory has become one of the accepted models of personality and as such is viewed as comprehensive and empirical within the field of personality psychology. Research on personality traits and their relation to health has begun to emerge, with the pace of research increasing because of the acceptance by researchers of the Big Five trait theory. This wide acceptance has also allowed researchers to be consistent when measuring personality traits and exploring the links between personality and health outcomes. For example, researchers have shown that higher levels of neuroticism can lead to an earlier death. People who are high in this particular trait are prone to worrying and anxiety, and becoming easily stressed, which in turn can lead to maladaptive coping methods such as smoking, drinking alcohol and taking illicit drugs, which have added health implications. Neuroticism also tends to be associated with a strong reaction to stressors, which can lead to physical illness (Van Heck, 1997). It is also reported that emotional instability associated with high levels of neuroticism is associated negatively with physical health and well-being (Hayes and Joseph, 2003). Conversely, extraversion, conscientiousness, agreeableness and openness have been found to be positively related to health and well-being. People's perception of health also appears to be affected by personality, with neuroticism reporting higher levels of health-care contact and poorer perceived health (Jerram and Coleman, 1999). Interestingly, for those high in neuroticism, higher levels of health-care contact may also lead to positive health outcomes because illnesses are detected and treated earlier.

Activity 9.4 — *Reflection*

Try the simple personality test in Table 9.1. Answer each question and score yourself against each of the 'Big Five' domains. On each question score as follows.

Strongly agree	4	Disagree	1
Agree	3	Strongly disagree	0
Neither agree or disagree	2		

Once you have finished, add your numbers together for each domain. Scores of 0–4 indicate low levels of that trait, scores of 4–8 indicate moderate levels and scores of 8–12 indicate high levels.

	Score
OPENNESS I have a vivid imagination. I have excellent ideas. I'm an adventurous person. TOTAL	
CONSCIENTIOUSNESS I am always prepared. I follow a schedule. I like order. TOTAL	
EXTRAVERSION I'm the life of the party. I don't mind being the centre of attention. I talk a lot to different people at parties. TOTAL	
AGREEABLENESS I'm soft hearted. I take time out for others. I empathise with others' feelings. TOTAL	
NEUROTICISM I get stressed out easily. I am easily irritated. I worry about things. TOTAL	

Table 9.1: Personality test

continued overleaf . . .

continued . . .

Remember that this test is for fun and will give you only a general idea of your score for each domain of personality type. Alternatively, complete the Big Five personality test by following the link: **www.outofservice.com/bigfive/**.

Does it reflect your personality? Compare your results with a friend.

As this is an individual activity, there is no outline answer at the end of the chapter.

A useful model that is common within the field of mental health nursing uses a framework that encapsulates concepts of stress and vulnerability, and is known as the stress vulnerability model (Zubin and Spring, 1977). The model suggests that vulnerability will result in the development of distress only when environmental stresses are present. If the vulnerability is high, fairly low levels of environmental stress might be enough to cause mental distress. If the vulnerability is low or you are more robust, mental distress will occur when higher levels of environmental stress are experienced. The stress vulnerability model seeks to define why certain individuals develop problems and others appear not to, even when they experience the same levels of stress or major life events. What is positive about this model is that although your vulnerability to stress may be fixed to a certain degree, it is possible to modify or manage the stress experienced and therefore reduce the impact on your health.

Adaptive and maladaptive coping

When faced with stress, individuals employ what are called coping strategies. These strategies can be viewed as either adaptive or maladaptive, or as positive and negative coping. If you think back to the *Five Ways to Well-being* or the five fruit and veg of mental health, these can be viewed as positive coping strategies with regard to stress. But what is negative coping? Negative coping can be seen as a strategy that briefly ameliorates the feelings of stress or mental distress but in the long term is likely to intensify the stress or distress felt (see Table 9.2).

The list in Table 9.2 is not exhaustive, and we all employ a variety of coping methods to deal with stress. What is important is to look at the ways you cope with stress and build upon your positive coping strategies while reducing the negative ways you may be coping with stress and in the long run adding to your stress. For more helpful and useful ways to manage and cope positively with stress, visit Mind Tools (see 'Useful websites' at the end of the chapter).

Much recent attention has been paid by some NHS Trusts and voluntary organisations to the idea of WRAP (Wellness and Recovery Action Planning). The goals of this approach are to teach people recovery and self-management skills and strategies for improving and managing their own mental health. The patient can choose to achieve this by working through WRAP individually, in groups or with the health-care professional.

WRAP is based on the work of Mary Ellen Copeland and represents an important way in which mental health nurses can enable and support the process of recovery. A key to this approach is

Positive coping	Negative coping
Maintain a healthy diet	Smoking
Write down thoughts and feelings	Illicit drugs
Confide in someone (seek emotional support)	Alcohol
Take exercise	Over-eating or under-eating
Practise relaxation or meditation techniques (be mindful)	Procrastinating, rumination
Participate in social events, hobbies, etc.	Avoidance
Resolve conflicts with others	Sleeping too much
Get enough sleep	Isolating, avoiding family and friends
Approach challenges as positive and not as a threat	Drinking too much caffeine

Table 9.2: Positive and negative coping

to plan ahead – to be aware of one's own needs and have an action and crisis plan in the event of problems arising. The approach is explicitly built on the idea of recovery. WRAP emphasises holistic health, wellness, strengths and social support (Cook et al., 2009).

WRAP is not just for those individuals who suffer with mental illness; people with all kinds of health conditions and even those who have no significant complaints but want to stay healthy have found WRAP to be useful. This is also true for those who want to make positive changes in the way they feel, increase their enjoyment in life or reduce the impact of stress (Copeland, 1997). Key aspects of WRAP include:

* wellness toolbox;
* daily maintenance plan;
* identifying triggers and an action plan;
* identifying early warning signs and an action plan;
* identifying when things are breaking down and an action plan;
* crisis planning;
* post-crisis planning.

If you consider the topics we have covered in this chapter, the strategies you can employ to improve your own well-being, protect yourself from the damaging effects of stress and therefore protect yourself from mental illness, then WRAP is a system you can use to draw together these strategies into one coherent system.

You may also like to start your own wellness toolbox for keeping yourself mentally healthy at work.

Chapter summary

In this chapter we have examined the historical context of health and well-being and how these concepts have changed over time. We have examined the links between the mind and body and how the Western world lost this concept of holism, the treatment of the whole person when approaching ill health. We discussed how and when the concept of holism began to reappear and looked at the distinction in health-care provision and how contemporary health care still exists within specific fields. We considered stress and its impact on health and how we can employ strategies in our day-to-day lives to enhance our well-being and protect ourselves from the damaging effects of stress. You were encouraged to think further about applying these ideas when considering the treatment of those with physical and mental ill health and how these approaches will enhance your skills in the holistic care of patients.

Activities: brief outline answers

Activity 9.1: Reflection (page 165)

When thinking of Dorothy's overall health you would also consider the wider determinants of health. With Dorothy you may look to address her physical environment at home, her benefits, income and her social support networks as well as her physical needs. This approach would require multi-agency working, which may involve contacting Dorothy's social worker who could arrange to have the physical environment attended to, benefit entitlement claimed and the development of social participation and the facilitation of a social network. This approach would place Dorothy at the centre of her care and would include working collaboratively with Dorothy to gain consent and her view of her problems and goals.

Activity 9.2: Reflection (page 166)

Further physical sensations you may experience when you feel nervous or anxious can be dependent on the individual and may range from the mild to the extreme. Some examples of these sensations may include:

- heart palpitations;
- trembling or shaking;
- breathlessness;
- difficulty swallowing;
- chest pain;
- nausea and vomiting;
- dizziness;
- hot and cold flushes;
- fear of losing control or 'going mad'.

Activity 9.3: Reflection (page 172)

You would want to consider if Jim understood the concepts of holism and how the biopsychosocial domains affect health and interact with one another. Perhaps you could offer Jim some education around this and explain the concept of stress and what he may do to protect himself from stress and its negative impact on mental health, well-being and physical health. Jim could be gently encouraged to first open his curtains to allow some natural light into his flat and gradually to increase his time spent out of the flat. You could even consider accompanying Jim on his first ventures out and encourage him to begin visiting the local Roman Catholic Church for mass or accompanying Jim on the bus to visit the local amenities. While Jim is at the local amenities he may be gently prompted to consider buying himself some ingredients to prepare himself a nutritious meal when he gets home. Again, you would consider offering Jim some education around the positive benefits of a healthy diet on his physical health and how this could improve his mental health and well-being. Eventually Jim could begin to think about getting in touch with his family. All of this would need to be planned carefully, not rushed, and taken in small achievable steps. You wouldn't want to move too fast in case Jim couldn't manage and then felt that he had failed in some way. You would also have to consider helping Jim with practical issues such as applying for a bus pass and planning his days, slowly building up his activity and confidence.

Further reading

Copeland, ME (1997) WRAP: Wellness Recovery Action Plan. Brattleboro, VT: Peach Press.

Using this framework, you can utilize a useful approach to overcoming distressing symptoms of mental illness, unhelpful behaviour patterns and developing ways of coping.

Foresight Mental Capital and Wellbeing Project (2008) Final project report: executive summary. London. The Government Office for Science.

This is a comprehensive, detailed and evidence-based resource on factors that influence an individual's mental development and well-being from conception until death.

Van de Weller, C (2005) Changing diets, changing minds: how food affects mental well being and behaviour, in Longfield, J, Ryrie, I and Cornah, D (eds) *Feeding minds: the impact of food on mental health*. London: Sustain, Mental Health Foundation and Food Commission.

This offers a comprehensive, detailed and evidence-based resource on how diet affects our mental well-being and behaviour, and how our diets have changed over the years.

Useful websites

www.mindtools.com/smpage.html

www.mindfulemployer.net/Feeling%20Stressed%20-%20Keeping%20Well.pdf

For helpful and useful ways to manage and cope positively with stress.

www.mentalhealth.org.uk/publications/feeding-minds-exec-summary/

For more detail and information on nutrition, well-being and health.

www.mentalhealth.org.uk/publications/be-mindful-report/

www.mentalhealth.org.uk/publications/be-mindful-toolkit/

For more information on the evidence for mindfulness approaches and its application.

www.outofservice.com/bigfive/

For more information on personality traits and accurate personality trait assessment scales.

www.mind.org.uk/foodandmood/food_and_mood-the_mind_guide#Which foods

For a comprehensive and detailed link between nutrition and mental health.

Glossary

ABV (alcohol by volume)   the standard measure of how much alcohol is contained in an alcoholic drink.

adaptive   responding in a helpful way/good coping

adrenaline   hormone and neurotransmitter that increases heart rate, contracts blood vessels and dilates air passages.

aetiology   the origins or causes of an illness or health issue.

amino acids   building blocks of proteins.

attending   the physical demonstration that you are interested and ready to listen.

behaviourism   a learning theory that suggests that human behaviour results from conditioning.

biopsychosocial model   a model that examines the biological, psychological and social aspects of health and illness.

cardiotoxic   having a harmful effect on the heart.

clarification   checking with the patient that you are understanding their experience (what they describe to you) correctly.

classical conditioning   a form of learning that stems from the work of Ivan Pavlov where a neutral stimulus becomes associated with another stimulus to produce a similar response.

clinical supervision   *a formal process of professional support and learning that enables individual practitioners to develop knowledge and competence, assume responsibility for their own practice and enhance consumer protection and safety of care in complex clinical situations* (DH, 1993).

cognition   the mental process of knowing and thinking and the way in which people think.

co-morbid mental distress   mental distress that exists at the same time as other health issues.

complete recovery   a cure for an illness or disorder; complete abatement of symptoms.

compliance   a willingness to adhere to medical treatment.

cortisol   steroid hormone produced by the adrenal gland.

counter-transference   the effect that transference has on a person and how they respond as a result (see also transference).

delusional   having a fixed and false belief that is not influenced by reasoned argument.

dementia   a serious reduction in cognitive ability that is greater than the normal ageing process.

ethical framework   the use of ethical guidelines to solve ethical dilemmas.

exploitation phase   the third of the phases of Peplau's interpersonal relations model concerned with when the patient begins to benefit from the nurse–patient relationship.

feedback   the giving or receiving of a person's thoughts on that of another, for example, how clearly a speech was made at a wedding, how funny it was.

funnelling   a style used when communicating with patients, starting with open questions and funnelling down to more specific questions.

holistic   taking a wide view of a situation or an individual and recognising the importance of the relationship between the parts of the situation or individual.

identification phase   the second of the phases of Peplau's interpersonal relations model concerned with when the patient begins to feel secure within and optimistic about the nurse–patient relationship.

individualism   belief in placing the individual first over that of the wider society or social group.

labelling   in sociology, the process of describing a person to identify aberrant behaviour.

leucine   essential amino acid that is not synthesised in the body but has to be obtained through food.

lysine   essential amino acid that is not synthesised in the body but has to be obtained through food.

maladaptive   responding in an unhelpful way/poor coping.

mindfulness   meditation based on Buddhist principles that is increasingly used in psychology and psychiatry to reduce the distressing nature of psychiatric symptoms. Some other applications for mindfulness include stress reduction, pain management and enhancing well-being.

mood   a state of feeling.

negative automatic thoughts   negative thinking about self, the world or the future that occur to a person seemingly without prior thought.

negative reinforcement   removal of an unpleasant stimulus to increase the occurrence of a behaviour.

neurons   cells that are found in the brain in vast numbers – estimates suggest 100 billion – that communicate with each other via electrical and chemical mechanisms.

neurosciences   the scientific study of the nervous system.

neurotransmitters   chemicals that transmit signals between neurons.

operant conditioning   a form of conditioning where the reinforcement of a behaviour influences its occurrence.

orientation phase   the first of the phases of Peplau's interpersonal relations model concerned with the initial stages of the nurse–patient relationship.

paranoid   a state where your thinking is governed by irrational fears.

perception   the way in which we detect and make sense of sensory information.

perceptual filtering   the way we filter stimuli (e.g., someone talking to us, reading a magazine) and then make sense out of it.

phenylalanine   essential amino acid that is not synthesised in the body but has to be obtained through food.

plaintiff   the party who sues in a civil action.

positive reinforcement   reward for a behaviour, which increases its occurrence.

precursor   compound that participates in generating or synthesising another different compound.

problem-oriented assessments   assessments that focus on need, inability and deficits.

proteins   organic compounds made from amino acids.

psychodynamics   the study of what psychological factors underpin human behaviours – particularly the relationship between conscious and unconscious motivation.

psychoneuroimmunology   the study of the link between psychological function or processes and the nervous and immune systems.

resolution phase   the evaluation of progress of interventions within the therapeutic relationship to see if the original issues have been resolved with a view to ending the relationship.

schizophrenia   a serious mental illness with psychotic features such as thought disorder, delusion and hallucinations.

self-actualisation   a psychological term for reaching your full potential in every area of your being – often a quest rather than a reality.

serious mental illness (SMI)   mental illnesses that include a diagnosis that typically involves psychosis and may require high levels of care and that may require hospital treatment. Typical examples of SMI include schizophrenia and bipolar disorder.

social recovery   a return to effective social functioning.

summarising   a way of demonstrating that you are actively listening by summarising what a patient has told you in a clear, concise way.

termination phase   the ending of the therapeutic relationship.

transference   occurs when a person takes the perceptions and expectations of one person and projects them on to another person.

tryptophan   essential amino acid that is not synthesised in the body but has to be obtained through food.

unconditional positive regard   the suspension of any form of personal judgement, and acceptance of the client regardless of the content of any disclosure they may have made.

References

Action for Advocacy (2002) *Advocacy Charter*. Available at: www.actionforadvocacy.org.uk (accessed 24 October 2010).

Adair, J (1997) *Decision-making and problem solving*. London: Institute of Personnel and Development.

Aked, J, Marks, N, Cordon, C and Thompson, S (2008) *Five Ways to Well-being: the evidence*. London: Government Office for Science, Foresight Project.

Anstiss, T and Bromley, P (2010) Exercise, in Margereson, C and Trenoweth, S (eds) *Developing holistic care for long-term conditions*. London: Routledge.

APA (American Psychiatric Association) (2000) *Diagnostic and statistical manual of mental disorders* (4th edn, text revision). Washington, DC: APA Publishing.

Arkowitz, H, Westra, HA, Miller, WR and Rollnick, S (eds) (2008) *Motivational interviewing in the treatment of psychological problems*. New York: Guilford Press.

Aveyard, H (2002) Implied consent prior to nursing care procedures. *Journal of Advanced Nursing*, July, 39 (2): 201–7.

Barker, P (2004) Assessment in psychiatric and mental health nursing, 2nd edn. Cheltenham: Nelson Thornes.

Baron-Cohen, S (2003) *The essential difference: the truth about the male and female brain*. New York: Basic Books, p21.

Beauchamp T and Childress J (2001) *Principles of biomedical ethics*, 5th edn. Oxford: Oxford University Press.

Beck, A (1976) *Cognitive therapy and the emotional disorders*. New York: International University Press.

Beck, W, van der Maesen, L and Walker, A (eds) (1997) *The social quality of Europe*. The Hague: Kluwer Law International.

Bennett, J (2008) Supporting recovery: medication management in mental health care, in Lynch, J and Trenoweth, S (eds) *Contemporary issues in mental health nursing*. Chichester: Wiley.

Bennett, JA, Lyons, KS, Winters-Stone, K, Nail, LM and Scherer, J (2007) Motivational interviewing to increase physical activity in long-term cancer survivors: a randomized controlled trial. *Nursing Research*, 56: 18–27. doi:10.1097/00006199–200701000–00003.

Bentall, R (2003) *Madness explained: psychosis and human nature*. London: Penguin.

Bessant, M, King, EA and Peveler, R (2008) Characteristics of suicides in recent contact with NHS Direct. *Psychiatric Bulletin*, 32: 92–5.

Blane, D (1991) Health profession. In Scambler, G (ed) *Sociology as applied to medicine*, 3rd edn, p213.

Bope, ET, Douglass, AB and Gibovsky, A (2004) Pain management by the family physician: the Family Practice Pain Education Project. *The Journal of the American Board of Family Medicine*, 17: S1–12.

Bowers L, Brennan G and Winship, G (2009) Talking with acutely psychotic people: communication skills for nurses and others spending time with people who are very mentally ill. London: City University. Available at: www.acutecareprogramme.org.uk/silo/files/talking-with-acutely-psychotic-people.pdf (accessed 12 September 2010).

Brown, A. (2006) Prenatal infection as a risk factor for schizophrenia, *Schizophrenia Bulletin*, 32 (2): 200–2.

Brown, G and Harris, T (1978) *The social origins of depression: a study of psychiatric disorder in women*. London: Tavistock.

Brown, M (2004) *Coping with depression after traumatic brain injury*. Available at www.adap.net/tbi/depression.pdf.

Brown, S, Birtwistle, J, Roe, L and Thompson, C (1999) The unhealthy lifestyle of people with schizophrenia. *Psychological Medicine*, 29 (3): 697–701.

Butcher, J, Mineka, S and Hooley, J (2008) *Abnormal psychology: core concepts*. Boston, MA: Pearson.

Carels, RA, Darby, L, Cacciapaglia, HM, Konrad, K, Coit, C, Harper, J et al. (2007) Using motivational interviewing as a supplement to obesity treatment: a stepped-care approach. *Health Psychology*, 26: 369–74. doi:10.1037/0278–6133.

Carney, RM, Rich, MW, Freedland, KE et al. (1988) Depressive disorder predicts cardiac events in patients with coronary artery disease. *Psychosomatic Medicine*, 50, 627–633.

Carr, A (2004) *Positive psychology*. Hove: Routledge.

Centre for Mental Health (2010) *The economic and social costs of mental health problems in 2009/10*. Available at: www.centreformentalhealth.org.uk/pdfs/Economic_and_social_costs_2010.pdf.

Chambers, C and Ryder, E (2009) *Compassion and caring in nursing*. Oxford: Radcliffe Publishing.

Channon, SJ, Huws-Thomas, MV, Rollnick, S, Hood, K, Cannings-John, RL, Rogers, C et al. (2007) A multicenter randomized controlled trial of motivational interviewing in teenagers with diabetes. *Diabetes Care*, 30: 1390–5. doi:10.2337/dc06–2260

Christensen, H, Low, L and Anstey, K (2006) Prevalence, risk factors and treatment for substance abuse in older adults. *Current Opinion in Psychiatry*, 19: 587–92.

Churchill, S (2011) *The troubled mind: a handbook of therapeutic approaches to psychological distress*. London: Palgrave Macmillan.

Ciechanowski, PS, Katon, WJ and Russo, JE (2000) Depression and diabetes: impact of depressive symptoms on adherence, function and costs. *Archives of Internal Medicine*, 160 (21): 3278–85.

Citrome, L and Yeomans, D (2005) Do guidelines for severe mental illness promote physical health and well-Being? *Journal of Psychopharmacology*, 19 (6): 102–9.

Clarkson, P (2003) *The therapeutic relationship*, 2nd edn. London: Whurr Publishers.

Collins dictionary (2001) 21st Century Edition. London: HarperCollins Publishers.

Cook, S (1999) The Self in self-awareness. *Journal of Advanced Nursing*, 29 (6): 1292–9.

Cook, J, Copeland, M, Hamilton, M, Jonikas, J, Razzano, L, Floyd, C, Hudson, W, Macfarlane, T and Grey, D (2009) Initial outcomes of a mental illness self-management program based on wellness recovery action planning. *American Psychiatric Association*, 60: 246–9.

Cooperman, NA, Parsons, JT, Chabon, B, Berg, KM and Arnsten, JH (2007) The development and feasibility of an intervention to improve HAART adherence among HIV-positive patients receiving primary care in methadone clinics. *Journal of HIV/AIDS and Social Services*, 6: 101–20. doi:10.1300/J187v06n01_07.

Copeland, ME (1997) *WRAP: Wellness Recovery Action Plan*. Brattleboro, VT: Peach Press.

Corrigan, PW and Phelan, SM (2004) Social support and recovery in people with serious mental illnesses. *Community Mental Health Journal*, 40: 513–23.

CSIP (Care Services Improvement Partnership) (2006) *Crisis resolution and home treatment: report from a conference linking research, policy and practice for service development* (5 October). Available at: www.acutecareprogramme.org.uk/silo/files/crisis-resolution-and-home-treatment.pdf.

Curtice, M and Exworthy, T (2009) FREDA: principles for a human rights based approach to healthcare. *Psychiatric Bulletin*, 16: 773–5.

Cutcliffe, JR and Barker, P (2004) The Nurses' Global Assessment of Suicide Risk (NGASR): developing a tool for clinical practice. *Journal of Psychiatric and Mental Health Nursing*, 11: 393–400.

Cutcliffe JR and Grant G (2001) What are the principles and processes of inspiring hope in cognitively impaired older adults within a continuing care environment? *Journal of Psychiatric and Mental Health Nursing*, 8: 427–36.

Daley, AJ (2002) Exercise therapy and mental health in clinical populations: is exercise therapy a worthwhile intervention? *Advances in Psychiatric Treatment*, 8: 262–70.

Dawson, J and Szmukler, G (2006) Fusion of mental health and incapacity legislation. *British Journal of Psychiatry*, 188 (6): 504–9.

Dean J, Todd G, Morrow H and Sheldon K (2001) Mum, I used to be good looking . . . look at me now: the physical health needs of adults with mental health problems: the perspectives of users, carers and front-line staff. *International Journal of Mental Health Promotion*, 3 (4): 16–24.

Delgado, P, Charney, D, Price, L, Aghajanian, G, Landis, H and Heninger, G (1990) Serotonin function and the mechanism of antidepressant action: reversal of antidepressant-induced remission by rapid depletion of plasma tryptophan. *Archives of General Psychiatry*, 47 (5): 411–18.

Department of Health and Human Services and Centres for Disease Control and Prevention (1996) *Physical activity and health: a report of the Surgeon General*. Atlanta, GA: Department of Health.

DH (Department of Health) (1993) *A vision for the future: report of the Chief Nursing Officer*. London: HMSO.

DH (1994) *Working in partnership: a collaborative approach to care* (report of the Mental Health Nursing Review Team). London: HMSO.

DH) (1997) *The new NHS: modern, dependable*. Available at: www.dh.gov.uk/en/Publicationsandstatistics/Publications/PublicationsPolicyAndGuidance/DH_4008869.

DH (1999a) *Saving lives: our healthier nation*. London: DH.

DH (1999b) *National Service Framework for Mental Health: modern standards and service models*. Available at: www.dh.gov.uk/en/Publicationsandstatistics/Publications/PublicationsPolicyAndGuidance/DH_4009598

DH (2000) *No secrets: guidance on developing and implementing multi-agency policies and procedures to protect vulnerable adults from abuse*. Available at: www.dh.gov.uk/en/Publicationsandstatistics/Publications/PublicationsPolicyAndGuidance/DH_4008486.

DH (2001a) *The expert patient: a new approach to chronic disease management for the 21st century*. Available at: www.dh.gov.uk/en/Publicationsandstatistics/Publications/PublicationsPolicyandGuidance/DH_4006801.

DH (2001b) *The mental health policy implementation guide*. London: Department of Health.

DH (2002) *National suicide prevention strategy for England*. Available at: www.dh.gov.uk/en/Publicationsandstatistics/Publications/PublicationsPolicyAndGuidance/DH_4009474.

DH (2004a) *Choosing health: making healthy choices easier*. Available at: www.dh.gov.uk/en/Publicationsandstatistics/Publications/PublicationsPolicyAndGuidance/DH_4094550.

DH (2004b) *At least five a week: evidence of the impact of physical activity and its relationship to health: a report from the Chief Medical Officer*. London: DH.

DH (2004c) *5 A Day*. Available at: www.dh.gov.uk/en/Publichealth/Healthimprovement/FiveADay/DH_4069867.

DH (2005) Mental Capacity Act 2005. Available at: http://webarchive.nationalarchives.gov.uk/+/www.dh.gov.uk/en/SocialCare/Deliveringadultsocialcare/MentalCapacity/MentalCapacityAct2005/index.htm.

DH (2006a) *Choosing health: supporting the physical needs of people with severe mental illness commissioning framework.* London: DH Publication.

DH (2006b) *From values to action: the Chief Nursing Officer's review of mental health nursing.* London: DH Publication.

DH (2008) *Refocusing care programme approach.* Available at: www.dh.gov.uk/en/Publicationsandstatistics/Publications/PublicationsPolicyAndGuidance/DH_083647.

DH (2009a) *New horizons: confident communities, brighter futures: a framework for developing well-being.* London: HM Government.

DH (2009b) *Reference guide to consent for examination or treatment*, 2nd edn. Available at: www.dh.gov.uk (accessed 20 November 2010).

DH (2010) *Equity and excellence: liberating the NHS.* Available at: www.dh.gov.uk/en/Publicationsandstatistics/Publications/PublicationsPolicyAndGuidance/DH_117353.

DH (2011a) *No health without mental health.* Available at: www.dh.gov.uk/en/Aboutus/Features/DH_123998.

DH (2011b) *Safeguarding adults: the role of health service practitioners.* Available at: www.dh.gov.uk (accessed 2 April 2011).

Dickson, D and Hargie, O (2006) Questioning, in Hargie, O (ed) *The handbook of communication skills.* London: Routledge, pp121–46.

Diener, E (1979) Deindividuation, self-awareness, and disinhibition, *Journal of Personality and Social Psychology*, 37 (7): 1160–71.

Diener, E and Seligman, MEP (2002) Very happy people. *Psychological Science*, 13: 81–4.

Dimond, B (2008) *Legal aspects of nursing*, 5th edn. Harlow: Pearson.

DRC (Disability Rights Commission) (2006) *Equal treatment, closing the gap: background evidence for the DRC's formal investigation into health inequalities experienced by people with learning disabilities and/or mental health problems.* Leeds: University of Leeds.

Duffy, T (1994) *Brief interventions and their role in relation to more intensive treatment of alcohol problems.* Addictions Update. Glasgow: Health Promotion Department, Greater Glasgow Health Board.

Duffy, T, Martin, C and Anstiss, T (2010) Facilitating, supporting and maintaining recovery, in Margereson, C and Trenoweth, S (eds) *Developing holistic care for long term conditions.* London: Routledge.

Durkheim, Emile (1997) [1951] *Suicide: a study in sociology.* New York: The Free Press.

Edwards, S. (2009) *Nursing ethics: a principle based approach*, 2nd edn. Basingstoke: Palgrave Macmillan.

Egan, G. (2010) *The skilled helper: a problem-management and opportunity development approach to helping*, 9th edn. London: Brookes/Cole CENGAGE Learning.

Engel, G (1977) The need for a new medical model. *Science*, 196: 129–36.

Ershler, W and Keller, E (2000) Age-associated increased Interleukin-6 gene expression, late life diseases and frailty. *Annual Review of Medicine*, 51: 245–70.

Etzioni A (1969) *The semi-professions and their organisation: teachers, nurses, social workers.* London: Collier Macmillan.

Faulkner, A and Layzell, S (2000) *Strategies for living: the research report.* London: Mental Health Foundation.

Faulkner, G and Sparkes, A (1999) Exercise therapy for schizophrenia: an ethnographic study. *Journal of Sport and Exercise*, 21: 39–51.

Feldman, HR (1981) A science of nursing: to be or not to be? *Image*, 13: 63–6.

Firn, M (2008) Engagement within the care planning process, in Hall, A, Kirby, S and Wren, M (eds) *Care planning in mental health: promoting recovery*. Oxford: Blackwell, p136–49.

Folkman, S (1992) Making the case for coping, in Carpenter, BN (ed) *Personal coping: theory, research and application* (pp 31–46). Westport, CN: Praeger Publishers.

Foresight Mental Capital and Wellbeing Project (2008) *Final project report: executive summary*. London. The Government Office for Science.

Fox, J and Gamble, C (2006) Consolidating the assessment process: the semi-structured interview, in Gamble, C and Brennan, G *Working with serious mental illness*, 2nd edn. Edinburgh: Elsevier.

Fredrickson, BL (2003) The value of positive emotions: the emerging science of positive psychology is coming to understand why it's good to feel good. *American Scientist*, 91: 330–5.

Freidmen, H and Silver, R (eds) (2007) *Foundations of health psychology*. New York: Oxford University Press.

Freud, S (2006) *The Penguin Freud reader*. London: Penguin.

Friedli, L and Dardis, C (2002) Smoke gets in their eyes. *Mental Health Today*, January: 18–21.

FSA (Food Standards Agency) (2001) *The balance of good health*. Available at: www.food.gov.uk/multimedia/pdfs/bghbooklet.pdf.

Future Vision Coalition (2009) *A future vision for mental health*. Available at: www.newvisionformentalhealth.org.uk/index.html.

Gamble, C (2006) Using low expressed emotion to develop positive therapeutic alliances, in: Gamble, C and Brennan, G (eds) *Working with serious mental illness: a manual for clinical practice*, 2nd edn. London: Elsevier, pp115–22.

Gilbert, P (2006) Evolution and depression: issues and implications. *Psychological Medicine*, 36: 287–97.

Gkika, S (2010) Helping anxious people, in Grant, A (ed) *Cognitive behavioural interventions for mental health practitioners*. Exeter: Learning Matters.

Goffman, E (1963) *Stigma*. Harmondsworth: Penguin.

Goldberg, D and Murray, R (2006) *The Maudsley handbook of practical psychiatry*, 5th edn. Oxford: Oxford University Press.

Goldberg, H (1977) *The hazards of being male: surviving the myth of masculine privilege*. New York: Signet Books.

Goldney, RD, Phillips, PJ, Fisher, LJ et al. (2004) Diabetes, depression and quality of life: a population study. *Diabetes Care*, 27 (5): 1066–70.

Good WJ (1960) Encroachment charlatanism and the emerging profession: psychiatry, sociology and medicine. *American Sociological Review*, 25: 902–14.

Goodman, B and Clemow, R (2008) *Nursing and working with other people*. Exeter: Learning Matters.

Gordon, R, Druckman, D, Rozelle, R and Baxter, J (2006) Non-verbal behaviour as communication, in Hargie, O (ed) *The handbook of communication skills*. London: Routledge, pp73–120.

Gough, S and Peveler, R (2004) Diabetes and its prevention: pragmatic solutions for people with schizophrenia. *British Journal of Psychiatry*, 184 (Suppl 47): S106–S111.

Griffiths, R (1983) *Report of the NHS Management Inquiry*. London: DHSS.

Grisso, T and Applebaum, PS (1995) The MacArthur Treatment Competence Study, III: abilities of patients to consent to psychiatric and medical treatments. *Law and Human Behaviour*, 19 (2): 149–74.

Gross, R (2010) Psychology: the science of mind and behaviour, 6th edn. London: Hodder.

Gureje, O (2007) Psychiatric aspects of pain. *Current Opinion in Psychiatry*, 20: 42–6.

Hackett, ML, Yapa, C, Parag, V et al. (2005) Frequency of depression after stroke: a systematic review of observational studies. *Stroke*, 36: 1330–40.

Halbreich, U and Palter, S. (1996) Accelerated osteoporosis in psychiatric patients: possible pathophysiological processes, *Schizophrenia Bulletin*, 22: 447–54.

Halbreich, U, Shen, J and Panaro, V (1996) Are chronic psychiatric patients at increased risk for developing breast cancer? *American Journal of Psychiatry*, 153: 559–60.

Hallahand, B and Garland, M (2005) Essential fatty acids and mental health. *The British Journal of Psychiatry*, 186: 275–7.

Haralambos, M and Holborn, M (2008) *Sociology: themes and perspectives*, 7th edn. Glasgow: Collins Educational.

Hargie, O (2006) *The handbook of communication skills*. London: Routledge.

Harris, E and Barraclough, B (1998) Excess mortality of mental disorder. *British Journal of Psychiatry*, 173: 11–53.

Hayes, N and Joseph, S (2003) Big 5 correlates of three measures of subjective well-being. *Personality and Individual Differences*, 34(4): 723–7.

HDA (Health Development Agency) (2002) *Manual for the Fast Alcohol Screen Test (FAST): fast screening for alcohol problems*. London: HDA. Available at: www.nice.org.uk.

Healthcare Commission (2006) *Variations in the experiences of patients using the NHS services in England*. London: Commission for Healthcare, Audit and Inspection.

Healy, D (2008) *Psychiatric drugs explained*. Oxford: Churchill Livingstone.

Healthcare Commission (2005) *Count me in: results of a national census of inpatients in mental health hospitals and facilities in England and Wales*. London: DH.

Hewitt, P (2005) Speech at the 'Britain speaks – effective public engagement and better decision making' conference. London, 23 June.

Holmes, T and Rahe, R (1967) The Social Readjustment Rating Scale. *Journal of Psychosomatic Research*, 11 (2): 213–18.

Horrobin, D (2001) *The madness of Adam & Eve*. Reading: Corgi Books.

Howard, LM, Kumar, C and Thornicroft, G (2002) The general fertility rate in women with psychotic disorders. *American Journal of Psychiatry*, 159 (6): 991–7.

Howard, S (2010) *Skills in psychodynamic counselling and psychotherapy*. London: Sage.

Howard League for Penal Reform (2005) *Briefing paper on prison overcrowding and suicide*. Available at: www.howardleague.org/suicides/.

Howatson-Jones, L (2010) *Reflective practice in nursing*. Exeter: Learning Matters.

Hoyle, E and John, P (1995) *Professional knowledge and professional practice*. London: Cassell.

Hunt. G. and Wainwright. P. (1994) *Expanding the role of the nurse*. Oxford: Blackwell Scientific Publications.

Huppert F (2008) *Psychological well-being: evidence regarding its causes and its consequences*. London: Foresight Mental Capital and Wellbeing Project.

Huxley, P and Thornicroft, G (2003) Social inclusion, social quality and mental illness. *British Journal of Psychiatry*, 182: 289–90.

International Council of Nurses (2010) Definition of nursing. Available at: www.icn.ch/about-icn/icn-definition-of-nursing/ (accessed 14 May 2011).

Iveson, C (2002) Solution-focused brief therapy. *Advances in Psychiatric Treatment*, 8: 149–56.

Jasper, M (2003) *Beginning reflective practice*. Cheltenham: Nelson Thornes.

Jenkins, R, Meltzer, H, Jones, P et al. (2008) *Foresight Mental Capital and Wellbeing Project. Mental health: future challenges*. London: The Government Office for Science.

Jerram, K and Coleman, P (1999) The Big Five personality traits and reporting of health problems and health behaviour in old age. *British Journal of Health Psychology*, 4 (2) 181–192.

Jones S, Howard L and Thornicroft G (2008) 'Diagnostic overshadowing': worse physical health care for people with mental illness. *Acta Psychiatr Scand*, September, 118 (3): 169–71.

Jugessur, T and Iles, IK (2009) Advocacy in mental health nursing: an integrative review of the literature. *Journal of Mental Health Nursing*, 16: 187–95.

Kagan, C and Evans, J (1995) *Professional interpersonal skills for nurses*. London: Chapman & Hall.

Kelly, C and McCreadie, RG (1999) Smoking habits, current symptoms and premorbid characteristics of schizophrenia patients in Nithsdale, Scotland. *American Journal of Psychiatry*, 156: 1751–7.

Kemp, P (2008) User involvement and the micro-politics of mental health care, in Lynch, J and Trenoweth, S (eds) *Contemporary issues in mental health nursing*. Chichester: Wiley.

Kendrick, T (1996) Cardiovascular and respiratory risk factors and symptoms among general practice patients with long-term mental illness. *British Journal of Psychiatry*, 169: 733–9.

Kessler, R, Berglund, P, Foster, C et al. (1997) Social consequences, psychiatric disorders, 11: Teenage Parenthood. *American Journal of Psychiatry*, 154: 1405–11.

Kolb, D (1984) *Experiential learning: experience as the source of learning and development*. Upper Saddle River, NJ: Prentice-Hall.

Koro, CE, Fedder, DO, L'italien, GJ et al. (2002) An assessment of the independent effects of olanzapine and risperidone exposure on the risk of hyperlipidaemia in schizophrenic patients. *Archive of General Psychiatry*, 59: 1021–6.

Kring, A, Johnson, S, Davison, G and Neale, J (2010) *Abnormal psychology*, 11th edn. Hoboken, NJ: Wiley.

Launer, J (2002) *Narrative-based primary care: a practical guide*. Abingdon: Radcliffe Medical Press.

Lavoie, KL, Bacon, SL, Barone, S et al. (2006) What is worse for asthma control and quality of life: depressive disorders, anxiety disorders, or both? *Chest*, 130: 1039–47.

Liaschenko, J and Peter, E (2004 Nursing ethics and conceptualisations of nurses: professional, practice and work. *Journal of Advanced Nursing*, 46 (5): 488–95.

Lyubomirsky, S, Sheldon, KM and Schkade, D (2005) Pursuing happiness: the architecture of sustainable change. *Review of General Psychology*, 9: 111–31.

Margereson, C and Trenoweth, S (eds) (2010) *Developing holistic care for long-term conditions*. London: Routledge.

Margereson, C, Trenoweth, S and Worledge, J (2010) Frameworks for comprehensive and holistic assessments, in Margereson, C and Trenoweth, S (eds) *Developing holistic care for long-term conditions*. London: Routledge.

Martin, G (1998) Ritual action and its effect on the role of the nurse as advocate. *Journal of Advanced Nursing*, 27, pp189–94.

Maslow, A. (1999) *Toward a psychology of being*, 3rd edn. New York: John Wiley & Sons.

Matthews, J (2008) The meaning of recovery, in Lynch, J and Trenoweth, S (eds) *Contemporary issues in mental health nursing*. Chichester: Wiley.

Matthews, J and Trenoweth, S (2008) Some considerations for mental health nurses working with patients who self-neglect, in Lynch, J and Trenoweth, S (eds) *Contemporary issues in mental health nursing*. Chichester: John Wiley and Sons.

McCabe, C (2002) Teaching assertiveness to undergraduate nursing students. *Nurse Education in Practice*, 3 (1): pp30–42.

McCabe, C and Timmins, F (2006) *Communication skills for nursing practice*. London: Palgrave Macmillan.

McCloughen, A (2003) The association between schizophrenia and cigarette smoking: a review of the literature and implications for mental health nursing practice. *International Journal of Mental Health Nursing*, 12: 119–29.

McCreadie, R (2003) Diet, smoking and cardiovascular risk in people with schizophrenia. *British Journal of Psychiatry*, 183: 534–9.

McLeod, J (1998) *An introduction to counselling*, 2nd edn. Buckingham: Open University Press.

McLeod, J (2007) *Counselling skills*. Maidenhead: McGraw Hill.

McManus, J, Pathansali, R, Stewart, R et al. (2007) Delirium post-stroke. *Age and Ageing*, 36: 613–18.

Mead, G (1934) *Mind, self and society*. Chicago, IL: University of Chicago Press.

Mental Health Foundation (2006) *Feeding minds: the impact of food on mental health*. Available at: www.mental health.org.uk/campaigns/food-and-mental-health/.

Mentality/NIMHE (2004) *Healthy body and mind: promoting health living for people who experience mental distress*. Available at: www.staffordshirementalhealth.info/ftp/document/pdf/shift-healthybody-workers.pdf.

Miller, WR and Rollnick, S (2002) *Motivational interviewing: preparing people for change*, 2nd edn. New York, Guilford Press.

Miller, WR and Rollnick, S (2009) Ten things that motivational interviewing is not. *Behavioural and Cognitive Psychotherapy*, 37: 129–40.

Morrison, V. and Bennett, P (2006) *An introduction to health psychology*. Harlow: Pearson.

Morrow, V (2001) *Networks and neighbourhoods: children's and young people's perspectives*. London: Health Development Agency.

Mosby's Medical, Nursing and Allied Health Dictionary (2000) 4th edn. Anderson, K (ed). St Louis, MO: Mosby.

Moss, B (2008) *Communication skills for health and social care*. London: Sage.

Mukherjee, S, Schnur, DB and Reddy, R (1989) Family history of type 2 diabetes in schizophrenic patients. *Lancet*, March 4, 1 (8636): 495.

Newman, A (2007) Self-concept in the nurse-client relationship, in Underman Boggs, K (ed) *Interpersonal relationships: professional communication skills for nurses*, 5th edn. St Louis, MO: Saunders Elsevier, pp64–90.

NHS ICHSC (National Health Information Centre) (2010) *In-patients formally detained in hospitals under the Mental Health Act 1983 and patients subject to supervised community treatment, Annual figures, England 2009/10*. Available at: www.ic.nhs.uk/statistics-and-data-collections/mental-health (accessed 4 February 2011).

NHSLA (National Health Service Litigation Authority) (2010) *Report and accounts.* Available at: www.nhsla.com (accessed 18 May 2011).

NHSLA (nd) *NHS indemnity: arrangements for handling clinical negligence claims against NHS staff* (DH HSG(96)48). Also the associated Good Practice document. Available at: www.nhsla.com in publications section (accessed 4 February 2011).

NICE (National Institute for Health and Clinical Excellence) (2006) *Dementia: supporting people with dementia and their carers in health and social care.* Available at: www.nice.org.uk/nicemedia/live/10998/30318/30318.pdf.

NICE (2007) *Depression (amended): management of depression in primary and secondary care.* Available at: www.nice.org.uk/Guidance/CG23.

NICE (2009a) *Medicines adherence.* Available at: www.nice.org.uk/guidance/index.jsp?action=download &o=43042.

NICE (2009b) *The treatment and management of depression in adults with chronic physical health problems.* Available at: http://guidance.nice.org.uk/CG91.

NICE (2009c) *Schizophrenia: core interventions in the treatment and management of schizophrenia in adults in primary and secondary care.* Available at: www.nice.org.uk/nicemedia/live/11786/43608/43608.pdf.

NIMHE (National Institute for Mental Health in England) (2005a) *Making it possible: improving mental health and well being in England.* London: Care Services Improvement Partnership. Available at: www.apho.org. uk/resource/view.aspx?RID=70037 (accessed 25 October 2010).

NIMHE (2005b) *NIMHE Guiding statement on recovery.* Available at: www.psychminded.co.uk/news/ news2005/feb05/nimherecovstatement.pdf.

NMC (Nursing and Midwifery Council) (2008a) *The code: standards of conduct, performance and ethics for nurses and midwives.* Available at: www.nmc-uk.org/Nurses-and-midwives/The-code/The-code-in-full/ (accessed 2 November 2010).

NMC (2008b) *Standards for medicines management.* Available at: www.nmc-uk.org/Documents/Standards/ nmcStandardsForMedicinesManagementBooklet.pdf.

NMC (2009) *Fitness for practice report 2009–10.* Available at: www.nmc-uk.org (accessed 2 December 2010).

NMC (2010a) *Standards for pre-registration nursing education.* Available at: http://standards.nmc-uk.org/ PublishedDocuments/Standards%20for%20pre-registration%20nursing%20education%2016082010.pdf.

NMC (2010b) *Guidance on professional conduct for nursing and midwifery students.* Available at: http://www.nmc-uk.org/Publications/Guidance/.

NMC (2010c) *What is fitness to practise?* Available at: www.nmc-uk.org/Hearings/What-is-fitness-to-practise.

Nolan, P and Badger, F (2005) Aspects of the relationship between doctors and depressed patients that enhance satisfaction with primary care. *Journal of Psychiatric and Mental Health Nursing*, 12: 146–53.

Nordqvist, C (2009) What is health? What does good health mean? Bexhill-on-Sea: MediLexicon International Ltd. Available at: www.medicalnewstoday.com/articles/150999.php (accessed 7 January 2011).

Novy, DM (2004) Psychological approaches for managing pain. *Journal of Psychopathology and Behavioural Assessment*, 26 (4): 279–88.

Nursing and Midwifery Order (2001). Available at: www.legislation.gov.uk/uksi/2002/253/contents/made (accessed 27 November 2010).

Nyanaponika, T (1972) *The power of mindfulness.* San Francisco, CA: Unity Press.

ODPM (Office of the Deputy Prime Minister) (2004) *Mental health and social exclusion: social exclusion unit report.* Wetherby: OPDM Publications.

Onega, L (1991) A theoretical framework for psychiatric nursing practice. *Journal of Advanced Nursing*, 16: 68–73.

ONS (Office for National Statistics) (2002) *The social and economic circumstances of adults with mental disorders.* London: TSO.

ONS (2011) *Suicide rates in the United Kingdom, 2000–2009.* Available at: www.statistics.gov.uk/pdfdir/sui0111.pdf.

Oxford English Reference Dictionary (1996) eds Pearsall, J and Trumble, B. New York: Oxford University Press, p481.

Peet, M (2004) Diet, diabetes and schizophrenia: review and hypothesis. *British Journal of Psychiatry*, 184 (Suppl 47): S102–S105.

Peplau, H (1988) *Interpersonal relations in nursing: a conceptual framework of reference for psychodynamic nursing.* New York: Springer.

Perna, R, Rouselle, A and Brennan, P (2003) Traumatic brain injury: depression, neurogenesis and medication management, *Journal of Head Trauma Rehabilation*, 18 (2): 201–3.

Phelan, M, Stradins, L and Morrison, S (2001) Physical health of people with severe mental illness. *British Medical Journal*, 322: 443–44.

Prochaska, JO and DiClemente, CC (1982) Transtheoretical theory: towards a more integrated model of change. *Psychotherapy: Theory, Research and Practice*, 19: 276–88.

Rau, J, Ehlebracht-Konig, I and Peterman, F (2008) Impact of a motivational intervention on coping with chronic pain: results of a controlled efficacy study. *Schmerz*, 22: 575–8, 580–5 (in German).

Raymont, V, Bingley, W, Buchanan, A, David, AS, Hayward, P and Wessely, S (2004) Prevalence of mental incapacity in medical inpatient and associated risk factors: cross sectional study. *Lancet*, 364 (9443): 1421–7.

RCN (Royal College of Nursing) (2003a) *Clinical supervision in the workplace: guidance for occupational health nurses.* London: RCN. Available at: www.rcn.org.uk/__data/assets/pdf_file/0007/78523/001549.pdf (accessed 18 September 2010).

RCN (2003b) *Defined nursing.* London: RCN. Available at: www.rcn.org.uk (accessed 10 December 2010).

RCP (Royal College of Physicians and Royal College of Psychiatrists) (1995) *Psychological care of medical patients: recognition and service provision: a joint working party report.* London: RCP.

Reeves, M and Orford, J (2002) *Fundamental aspects of legal, ethical and professional issues in nursing.* Salisbury: Mark Allen/Quay Books.

Repper, J (2000) Social inclusion, in Thompson, T and Mathias, P (eds) *Lyttle's mental health and disorder*, 3rd edn. London: Elsevier.

Repper, J and Perkins, R (2003) *Social inclusion and recovery: a model for mental health practice.* Edinburgh: Bailliere Tindall.

Repper, J and Perkins, R (2009) Challenging discrimination: promoting rights and citizenship, in Reynolds, J, Muston, R, Heller, T et al. (eds) *Mental health still matters.* Basingstoke: Palgrave.

Rethink (2005) *A report on the work of the recovery learning sites and other recovery-orientated activities and its incorporation into the Rethink Plan 2004–08.* Available at: www.rethink.org/document.rm?id=1042.

Rilling, J, Glenn, A, Jairam, M, Pagnoni, G, Goldsmith, D, Elfenbein, H and Lilienfeld, S (2007) Neural correlates of social cooperation and non-cooperation as a function of psychopathy. *Biological Psychiatry*, 61: 1260–71.

Robson, D and Gray, R (2005) Can we help people with schizophrenia stop smoking? *Mental Health Practice*, 9 (4): 14–18.

Robson, D and Gray, R (2007) Serious mental illness and physical health problems: a discussion paper. *International Journal of Nursing Studies*, 44: 457–66.

Robson, H, Margereson, C and Trenoweth, S (2008) Comorbidity in physical and mental ill health, in Lynch, J and Trenoweth, S (eds) *Contemporary issues in mental health nursing*. Chichester: Wiley.

Rogers, C (1951) *Client-centred therapy: its current practice, implications and theory*. Boston, MA: Houghton Mifflin.

Rogers, C (1959) A theory of therapy, personality and interpersonal relationships, as developed in the client-centered framework, in Koch, S (ed) *Psychology: a study of science. Vol. 3: Formulations of the person and the social context*. New York: McGraw Hill, pp210–11; 184–256.

Rogers, C (1961) *On becoming a person*. Boston, MA: Houghton Mifflin.

Rogers, C (1980) *A way of being*. Boston, MA: Houghton Mifflin.

Rose, D (2001) *Users' voices: perspectives of mental health service users on community and hospital care*. London: Sainsbury Centre for Mental Health.

Rosenhan, D (1973) On being sane in insane places. *Science*, 179 (January): 250–8.

Royal College of Psychiatry (2008) *Fair deal for mental health*. Available at: www.rcpsych.ac.uk.

Rumbold G (1999) *Ethics in nursing practice*. London: Elsevier Health Sciences.

Rungapadiachy, D (2008) *Self-awareness in healthcare: engaging in helping relationships*. Basingstoke: Palgrave Macmillan.

Ryan, MCM, Collins, P and Thakore, JH (2003) Impaired fasting glucose tolerance in first episode, drug naïve patients with schizophrenia. *American Journal of Psychiatry*, 159: 561–6.

Sabates, R and Hammond, C (2008) *The impact of lifelong learning on happiness and well-being*. London: Institute of Education.

Sanders, P (2003) *First steps in counselling: a student's companion for basic introductory courses*, 3rd edn. Ross-on-Wye: PCCS Books.

Schuller, T, Brasset-Grundy, A, Green, A, Hammond, C and Preston, J (2002) *Learning, continuity and change in adult life: wider benefits of learning research report*. London: Institute of Education.

Scottish Executive (2002) *Integrated care for drug users: assessments. Digest of tools used in the assessment process and core data sets*. Available at: www.drugmisuse.isdsscotland.org/eiu/intcare/intcare.htm.

Scottish Executive (2005) *Equal minds*. Available at: www.scotland.gov.uk/Publications/2005/11/0414 5113/51135.

Seligman, M. (2002) *Authentic happiness*. London: Nicholas Brearley Publishing.

Seligman, M. (2008) Positive health. *Applied Psychology: An International Review*, 57, 3–18.

Seymour, L (2003) *Not all in the mind: the physical health of mental health service users*. Briefing paper 2. London: Radical Mentalities.

Sheild, H, Fairbrother, G and Obmann, H (2005) Sexual health knowledge and risk behaviour in young people with first episode psychosis. *International Journal of Mental Health Nursing*, 14: 149–54.

Simmons, J and Griffiths, R (2009) *CBT for beginners*. London: Sage.

Simpson, A and Brennan, G (2009) Working in partnership, in Callaghan, P, Playle, J and Cooper, L (eds) *Mental health nursing skills*. Oxford: Oxford University Press, pp74–84.

Sin, J and Trenoweth, S (2010) Caring for the mind, in Margereson, C and Trenoweth, S (eds) *Developing holistic care for long term conditions*. London: Routledge.

Skinner, B. (1965) *Science and human behaviour*. New York: The Free Press.

Sleicher, LI (1981) Nursing is not a profession. *Nursing and Health Care*, 2 (4): 186–191, 218.

Snyder, C and Lopez, S (2005) *Handbook of positive psychology*. Oxford: Oxford University Press.

Social Exclusion Unit (2004) *Social exclusion and mental health*. London: ODPM.

Social Services Inspectorate (2002) *Modernising mental health services: inspection of mental health services*. London: Department of Health.

Spataro, J, Mullen, P, Burgess, P, Wells, D and Moss, S (2004) Impact of child sexual abuse on mental health. *The British Journal of Psychiatry*, 184: 416–21.

Stedman's Medical Dictionary (2000) 27th edn. Baltimore, MD: Lippincott William & Wilkins, p622.

Stein-Parbury, J. (2005) *Patient and person: interpersonal skills in nursing*, 3rd edn. Sydney: Elsevier Churchill Livingstone.

Stubbs, J and Gardner, L (2004) Survey of staff attitudes to smoking in a large psychiatric hospital. *Psychiatric Bulletin*, 28: 204–7.

Sullivan, HS (1968) *The interpersonal theory of psychiatry*. New York: W. W. Norton & Co.

Sullivan, J (2010) Helping people who hear voices and have false beliefs, in: Grant, A (ed) *Cognitive behavioural interventions for mental health practitioners*. Exeter: Learning Matters.

Swinton, J (2001) *Spirituality and mental health care: rediscovering a forgotten dimension*. London: Jessica Kingsley.

Thompson, I, Melia, K, Boyd, K and Horsburgh, D (2000) *Nursing ethics*, 4th edn. Oxford: Churchill Livingstone.

Thompson, I, Melia, K, Boyd, K and Horsburgh, D (2006) *Nursing ethics*, 5th edn. Oxford: Churchill Livingstone.

Thurgood, M (2009) Engaging clients in their care and treatment, in Norman, I and Ryrie, I (eds) *The art and science of mental health nursing: a textbook of principle and practice*, 2nd edn. Maidenhead: Open University Press, p621–36.

Tosevski, DL and Milovancevic, MP (2006) Stressful life events and physical health. *Current Opinion in Psychiatry*, 19: 184–9.

Trenoweth, S and Allymamod, W (2010) Mental health, in Margereson, C and Trenoweth, S (eds) *Developing holistic care for long term conditions*. London: Routledge.

Trenoweth, S and Lynch, J (2008) Masculinity as a risk variable in physical and mental ill health, in Lynch, J and Trenoweth, S (eds) *Contemporary issues in mental health nursing*. Chichester: Wiley.

Trenoweth, S and Price, I (2008) Truth, uncertainty and the mental health nurse, in Lynch, J and Trenoweth, S (eds) *Contemporary issues in mental health nursing*. Chichester: Wiley.

Trenoweth, S and Tobutt, C (2009) Assessing alcohol use and misuse in primary care, in Martin, C (ed) *Identification and treatment of alcohol dependency*. Cumbria: M&K Publishing.

Underman Boggs, K (2007a) Bridges and barriers in the therapeutic relationship, in Arnold, E and Underman Boggs, K (eds) *Interpersonal relationships: professional communication skills for nurses*, 5th edn. St Louis, MO: Saunders Elsevier, pp. 117–36.

Underman Boggs, K (2007b) Communication styles, in Arnold, E and Underman Boggs, K (eds) *Interpersonal relationships: professional communication skills for nurses*, 5th edn. St Louis, MO: Saunders Elsevier, pp185–98.

Underman Boggs, K (2007c) Resolving conflict between nurse and client, in Arnold, E and Underman Boggs, K (eds) *Interpersonal relationships: professional communication Skills for nurses*, 5th edn. St Louis, MO: Saunders Elsevier, pp318–38.

Van de Weyer, C (2005) Changing diets, changing minds: how food affects mental well being and behaviour, in Longfield, J, Ryrie, I and Cornah, D (eds) *Feeding minds: the impact of food on mental health*. London: Sustain, Mental Health Foundation and Food Commission.

Van Heck, G (1997) Personality and physical health: toward an ecological approach to health related personality research. *European Journal of Personality*, 11: 415–43.

Vanina, Y, Podolskaya, A, Sedky, K et al. (2002) Body weight changes associated with psychopharmacology. *Psychiatric Services*, 53 (7): 842–7.

Vanwormer, J and Boucher, JL (2004) Motivational interviewing and diet modification: a review of the evidence. *Diabetes Educator*, 30: 404–19.

Vose, CP (2000) Drug abuse and mental illness: psychiatry's next challenge! in Thompson, T and Mathias, P (eds) *Lyttle's mental health and disorder*, 3rd edn. London: Elsevier.

Warner, R. (1985) *Recovery from schizophrenia: psychiatry and political economy*. London: Routledge and Kegan Paul.

Watkins, CL, Auton, MF, Deans, CF, Dickinson, HA, Jack, CIA, Lightbody, CE et al. (2007) Motivational interviewing early after acute stroke: a randomized, controlled trial. *Stroke*, 38: 1004–9.

Watkins, P. (2001) *Mental health nursing: the art of compassionate care*. Edinburgh: Butterworth Heinemann.

Weinstein, J (2008) Promoting inclusivity in care planning, in Hall, A, Kirby, S and Wren, M (eds) *Care planning in mental health: promoting recovery*. Oxford: Blackwell, pp177–90.

WHO (World Health Organization) (1946) International Health Conference, New York, 19 June–22 July. Official Records of the World Health Organization, no. 2, p. 100. Geneva: WHO.

WHO (2004) *International statistical classification of diseases and related health problems, tenth revision (ICD-10)* Vol. 2. Geneva: WHO.

WHO (2010) *Mental health: strengthening our response*. Fact sheet No 220, WHO. Media Centre, WHO. Available at: www.who.int/mediacentre/factsheets/fs220/en/index.html (accessed 13 October 2010).

WHO (2011) *Health impact assessment: determinants of health*. Available at: www.who.int/hia/evidence/doh/en/.

Woodbridge, K and Fulford, B (2004) *Whose values? A workbook for values-based practice in mental health care*. London: Sainsbury Centre for Mental Health.

Wosket, V (2002) *The therapeutic use of self: counselling practice, research and supervision*. London: Routledge.

Zubin, J and Spring, B. (1977) Vulnerability: a new view of schizophrenia. *Journal of Abnormal Psychology*, 86 (2): 103–24.

Index